MAKE SMART CHOICES ABOUT THE FOODS YOU EAT AND PUT YOURSELF IN CHARGE WITH . . .

THE CORINNE T. NETZER 1997 CALORIE COUNTER

Counting calories is crucial when you're trying to lose weight and keep it off. You want to feel satisfied, but you don't want to exceed your daily caloric intake. So whether you're trying one of the newest brand-name foods, browsing the supermarket for something different, planning a night out at a fine restaurant, or composing a holiday feast, everything you need to know to make informed, healthful choices is right here, in this handy pocket guide.

Join the millions of weight-conscious consumers who have lost pounds and kept them off with Corinne T. Netzer's help. Discover the latest information about the newest foods, updated facts about old favorites, and much more in the book that gives you the knowledge you need to take control of your eating at last!

Books by Corinne T. Netzer:

THE CORINNE T. NETZER ANNUAL CALORIE COUNTER
THE BRAND-NAME CALORIE COUNTER
THE BRAND-NAME CARBOHYDRATE GRAM COUNTER
THE CHOLESTEROL CONTENT OF FOOD
THE COMPLETE BOOK OF FOOD COUNTS
THE CORINNE T. NETZER CALORIE COUNTER
THE CORINNE T. NETZER CARBOHYDRATE GRAM COUNTER
THE CORINNE T. NETZER DIETER'S DIARY
THE CORINNE T. NETZER ENCYCLOPEDIA OF FOOD VALUES
THE CORINNE T. NETZER FAT GRAM COUNTER
THE CORINNE T. NETZER FIBER COUNTER
THE CORINNE T. NETZER LOW-FAT DIARY
THE DIETER'S CALORIE COUNTER
THE COMPLETE BOOK OF VITAMIN & MINERAL COUNTS

THE COMPLETE BOOK OF FOOD COUNTS COOKBOOK SERIES:
100 LOW FAT SMALL MEAL AND SALAD RECIPES
100 LOW FAT VEGETABLE AND LEGUME RECIPES
100 LOW FAT SOUP AND STEW RECIPES
100 LOW FAT PASTA AND GRAIN RECIPES
100 LOW FAT FISH AND SHELLFISH RECIPES
100 LOW FAT CHICKEN AND TURKEY RECIPES

THE CORINNE T. NETZER 1997 CALORIE COUNTER

Corinne T. Netzer

A Dell Book

Published by
Dell Publishing
a division of
Bantam Doubleday Dell Publishing Group, Inc.
1540 Broadway
New York, New York 10036

ISBN: 0-440-22225-7

Printed in the United States of America

Published simultaneously in Canada

February 1997

10 9 8 7 6 5 4 3 2 1

Introduction

The Corinne T. Netzer Calorie Counter has been compiled with a twofold purpose: as an annual to keep you up-to-date with many of the changes made by the food industry, and to provide a slim, handy, put-in-purse-or-pocket volume.

My books *The Complete Book of Food Counts* and *The Brand-Name Calorie Counter* are much larger in size and scope, and are therefore much less portable. However, *THIS BOOK LISTS MORE PRODUCTS THAN ANY OTHER BOOK OF ITS SIZE!*

To keep this book concise yet comprehensive, I have grouped together listings of the same manufacturer whenever possible. Many brand-name yogurts, for example, are listed as "all flavors." Therefore, instead of three pages filled with individual flavors of yogurt, all with identical calorie counts, I have been able to use the extra space for many other products. And for many basic foods and beverages (such as butter, milk, and alcoholic beverages) I have used generic listings, rather than include the numerous brands with the same or similar caloric values.

Finally, in the process of updating this edition, it was necessary to eliminate many previous listings and brands to accommodate new products and different brands. If you do not find a specific brand-name food that was listed in a previous edition of this book, *this does not necessarily mean that the food product is no longer available.* Also, since food producers are constantly revising and improving products, the caloric counts of your favorite food may have changed even if the description of the product hasn't. Be sure to check for updated entries and to consult labels.

This book contains data from individual producers and manufacturers and from the United States government. It contains the most current information available as we go to press.

Good luck—and good eating.

C.T.N.

Abbreviations

approx.	approximately
diam.	diameter
fl.	fluid
lb.	pound(s)
oz.	ounce(s)
pkg.	package
pkt.	packet
tbsp.	tablespoon
tsp.	teaspoon

Symbols

″	inch
<	less than
*	prepared according to basic package directions

Note: Brand-name foods and restaurants listed in italics denote registered trade names.

A

FOOD AND MEASURE	CALORIES
Acerola, fresh, trimmed, ½ cup	16
Acorn squash:	
baked, cubed, ½ cup	57
boiled, mashed, ½ cup	41
Adzuki beans, dry (*Arrowhead Mills*), ¼ cup	160
Alfalfa sprouts, 1 cup:	
(*Arrowhead Mills*)	30
plain or with garlic or onion (*Jonathan's*)	25
Alfredo sauce:	
(*Ragu*), ¼ cup	110
(*Progresso*), ½ cup	300
three cheese (*Lawry's*), 3 tbsp.	70
refrigerated (*Contadina*), ½ cup	400
refrigerated (*Contadina* Light), ½ cup	190
Alfredo sauce mix:	
(*Knorr*), ⅓ pkg.	60
(*Spice Islands*), ½ pkg.	45
Alfredo seasoning mix (*Lawry's*), 1½ tbsp.	35
Allspice, 1 tsp.	.5
Almond, shelled:	
(*Dole*), 1 oz.	170
dried, dry-roasted, or honey-roasted, 1 oz.	167
dried, slivered, ¼ cup	200
oil-roasted, 1 oz.	176
slivered (*Planter's Gold Measure*), 2-oz. pkg.	340
Almond butter, crunchy or creamy (*Roaster Fresh*), 1 oz.	184
Almond paste (*Solo*), 2 tbsp.	180
Amaranth, boiled, drained, ½ cup	14
Anasazi beans (*Arrowhead Mills*), ¼ cup	150
Anchovy, canned, in olive oil, 5 medium, .7 oz.	42
Anchovy paste (*Reese*), 1 tbsp.	30
Angel hair pasta entree, frozen, 1 pkg.:	
(*Lean Cuisine*)	210

Angel hair pasta entree *(cont.)*
(*Smart Ones*) 170
with sausage (*Marie Callender's*) 370
Angel hair pasta mix, dry:
chicken (*Golden Saute*), ½ pkg. 210
Parmesan (*Golden Saute*), ½ pkg. 240
Anise seed, 1 tsp. 7
Apple:
fresh, with peel, 2¾" apple 81
fresh, with or without peel, sliced, ½ cup 32
canned, sliced (*White House*), ½ cup 100
dried (*Sonoma*), 10–12 pieces, 1.4 oz. 110
frozen, escalloped (*Stouffer's*), ½ of 12-oz. pkg. 180
spiced rings (*S&W*), 2 rings 25
Apple butter, 1 tbsp.:
(*Apple Time/Lucky Leaf/Musselman's*) 30
(*Smucker's/Simply Fruit*) 4
Apple drink blends, 8 fl. oz., except as noted:
all flavors except peach-kiwi and peach-plum (*Veryfine Quenchers*) 120
berry, frozen* (*Dole* Burst) 120
cranberry (*Dole*), 10 fl. oz. 160
peach-kiwi or peach-plum (*Veryfine Quenchers*) 130
raspberry (*Tree Top*), 10 fl. oz. 190
raspberry-blackberry (*Tropicana Twister*) 130
Apple fritters, frozen (*Mrs. Paul's*), 2 pieces 260
Apple juice, 8 fl. oz., except as noted:
(*Apple & Eve*) 110
(*Heinke's* Organic/Gravenstein) 120
(*Minute Maid*) 120
(*Musselman's* Regular/Natural/Premium/Cider) 120
(*Snapple* Crisp), 10 fl. oz. 140
frozen* (*Minute Maid*) 110
Apple juice blends, 8 fl. oz.:
all blends, except cherry cider (*R. W. Knudsen*) 120
apricot, cherry, or strawberry (*After the Fall*) 100
cherry cider (*R. W. Knudsen*) 130
cranberry (*Tree Top*) 130
grape, bottled or frozen* (*Tree Top*) 130

orange (*Tree Top* Fiber Rich) 170
pear (*Tree Top*) 120
raspberry (*After the Fall*) 90
raspberry (*Tree Top*) 110
Apple pastry (also see specific listings), 1 piece:
dumpling, frozen (*Pepperidge Farm*) 290
pocket (*Tastykake*) 380
squares, frozen (*Pepperidge Farm*) 210
Applesauce, ½ cup:
(*Musselman's* Chunky/Cinnamon) 100
(*S&W* Gravenstein) 90
unsweetened (*Lucky Leaf/Musselman's* Regular/
Cinnamon) 50
unsweetened (*S&W* Gravenstein) 50
Apricot:
fresh, 3 medium, 12 per lb. 51
canned, in juice (*Del Monte* Lite), ½ cup 60
canned, in heavy syrup (*S&W*), ½ cup 110
dried, Turkish (*Dole Sun Giant*), 1.4 oz., 6 pieces 90
Apricot nectar, 8 fl. oz. (*Libby's/Kern's*) 150
Arby's, 1 serving:
breakfast items:
bacon, 2 strips 90
biscuit, plain 280
blueberry muffin 230
cinnamon-nut danish 360
croissant, plain 220
egg portion 95
French-Toastix, 6 pieces 430
ham 45
sausage 163
table syrup 100
sandwiches:
chicken, breaded fillet 536
chicken, Cordon Bleu 623
chicken, grilled, deluxe 430
chicken, grilled, BBQ 388
chicken, roast, club 546
chicken, roast, deluxe, light 276

Arby's*, sandwiches *(cont.)

chicken, roast, deluxe, sesame seed bun 433
chicken, roast, Santa Fe 436
ham 'n cheese 359
ham 'n cheese melt 329
fish fillet 529
roast beef, *Arby's* Melt with cheddar 368
roast beef, *Arby-Q* 431
roast beef, Bac'n Cheddar deluxe 539
roast beef, Beef'n Cheddar 487
roast beef, deluxe, light 296
roast beef, giant 555
roast beef, junior 324
roast beef, regular 388
roast beef, super 523
roast turkey, deluxe, light 260

sandwiches, sub roll:

French dip 475
hot Ham 'n Swiss 500
Italian sub 675
Philly Beef 'n Swiss 755
roast beef sub 700
triple cheese melt 720
turkey sub 550

chicken fingers, 2 pieces 290

soups:

Boston clam chowder 190
broccoli, cream of 160
cheese, Wisconsin 280
chicken noodle 80
chili, Timberline 220
potato with bacon 170
vegetable, lumberjack 90

potatoes:

baked, plain• 355
baked, Broccoli 'n Cheddar 447
baked, deluxe 736
baked, with margarine and sour cream 578
cakes, 2 pieces 204

fries, curly 300
fries, cheddar curly 333
fries, french 246
salad, garden 61
salad, roast chicken 149
salad, side 23
sauces and dressings:
Arby's Sauce 15
barbecue sauce 30
beef stock au jus 10
blue cheese dressing 290
buttermilk ranch, reduced calorie 50
cheddar dressing 35
honey French dressing 280
honey mayonnaise, reduced calorie 70
Horsey Sauce 60
Italian dressing, reduced calorie 20
Italian sub or Parmesan sauce 70
ranch dressing, red 75
tartar sauce 140
Thousand Island dressing 260
desserts:
apple turnover 330
cheesecake, plain 320
cherry turnover 320
chocolate chip cookie 125
Polar Swirl Butterfinger 457
Polar Swirl Heath 543
Polar Swirl Oreo 482
Polar Swirl peanut butter cup 517
Polar Swirl Snickers 511
shake, chocolate 451
shake, jamocha 384
shake, vanilla 360
Arrowroot flour, 1 cup 457
Artichoke, globe (see also "Jerusalem artichoke"):
fresh, boiled, hearts, drained, ½ cup 42
canned, bottoms (*S&W*), 3 pieces 25
canned, hearts (*S&W*), 3 pieces 30

Artichoke ***(cont.)***
frozen, hearts, 9-oz. pkg. 96
marinated (*S&W*), 2 pieces, 1 oz. 30
Arugula, trimmed, 2 cups, 1 oz. 7
Asparagus:
fresh, boiled, 4 spears, ½″ diameter base 14
canned (*S&W* Blended), 6 pieces, 4.5 oz. 15
canned, spears, all varieties (*Green Giant/LeSueur*), 4.5 oz. 20
frozen (*Birds Eye*), 3 oz. 20
Atemoya (*Frieda's*), 3.5 oz. 94
Au jus gravy, ¼ cup:
canned (*Franco-American*) 10
mix* (*Knorr*) 15
Au jus seasoning mix (*Durkee/French's* Roasting Bag), ⅛ pkg. 10
Avocado, California, fresh:
1 medium, 8 oz. 306
pureed, ½ cup 204
Avocado dip (*Nalley*), 2 tbsp. 120

B

FOOD AND MEASURE	CALORIES
Bacon (see also "Turkey bacon"):	
(*Boar's Head*), 2 slices	60
(*Hormel* Microwave), 2 slices	70
(*John Morrell* Hardwood Smoked), 2 slices	100
(*Oscar Mayer* Regular/Lower Sodium), 2 slices	60
(*Oscar Mayer* 1/8" Thick), 1 slice	60
(*Oscar Mayer* Center Cut), 3 slices	90
(*Rock River/Sinnissippi*), 2 slices	80
(*Sweet Applewood Farms*), 2 slices	80
Bacon, Canadian:	
(*Boar's Head*), 2 oz.	70
(*Oscar Mayer*), 2 slices, 1.6 oz.	50
Bacon, Irish, back, 2 slices, 2 oz.	130
"Bacon," vegetarian (*Morningstar Farms*), 2 strips	60
Bacon bits:	
(*Oscar Mayer*), 1 tbsp.	25
imitation (*Bac*Os*), 1 tbsp.	30
Bacon dip:	
horseradish (*Heluva Good*), 2 tbsp.	60
onion (*Nalley*), 2 tbsp.	60
Bagel, 1 piece:	
egg or cinnamon raisin (*Thomas'*)	160
plain, onion, or multigrain (*Thomas'*)	150
plain or cinnamon raisin (*Awrey's*)	200
Bagel, frozen, cinnamon raisin (*Sara Lee*), 1 piece	220
Baked beans, 1/2 cup:	
(*Campbell's* New England/Old Fashioned)	180
(*Campbell's* Homestyle)	150
(*S&W* Brick Oven)	160
bacon and brown sugar (*Campbell's/Campbell's* Old Fashioned)	170
bacon and brown sugar or Texas-style barbecue (*S&W*)	140
barbecue (*Campbell's* Old Fashioned/Tangy)	170

Baked beans *(cont.)*
honey mustard (*S&W*) 130
maple sugar (*S&W*) 150
and pork (*Campbell's*) 130
and pork (*Stokely* Sugar) 150
and pork (*Stokely* Tomato) 140
and pork, with jalapeño (*Trappey's*) 130
and pork, with peas (*East Texas Fair* Peas 'n Pork) 110
vegetarian (*Campbell's*) 130
vegetarian (*Stokely*) 140
vegetarian, with brown sugar sauce (*Stokely*) 150
Baking mix, all purpose (*Arrowhead Mills*), 1/4 cup 140
Baking powder (*Davis*), 1 tsp. 8
Balsam pear, fresh:
leafy tips, boiled, drained, 1/2 cup 10
pods, boiled, drained, 1/2" pieces, 1/2 cup 12
Bamboo shoots:
boiled, drained, 1/2" slices, 1/2 cup 8
canned, drained (*La Choy*), 1/4 cup 5
Banana:
1 medium, 8 3/4" long 105
dried (*Sonoma*), 2 pieces, 1 1/2 oz. 140
Banana, manzano (*Frieda's*), 1 oz. 24
Banana, red, 1 medium, 7 1/4" long 118
Banana nectar, 11.5-fl.-oz. can:
(*Libby's/Kern's*) 190
blend (*Libby's* Quanabana) 210
blend, with pineapple (*Kern's*) 220
Banana squash, baked (*Frieda's*), 1 oz. 18
Barbecue dip (*Heluva* Good Rib-Ticklin'), 2 tbsp. 60
Barbecue sauce, 2 tbsp.:
(*Heinz* Thick & Rich Old Fashioned) 40
(*Hunt's* Original/Dijon Mild/Mild/Mesquite) 40
(*Hunt's* Original Bold) 45
(*KC Masterpiece* Original) .60
(*Lea & Perrins* Original/Bold & Spicy) 50
(*Open Pit* Original/Hickory Smoke/Hot/Mesquite/Sweet) . . .50
all varieties (*Healthy Choice*) 25
Buffalo wing (*Heinz*) 15

Cajun (*Luzianne*) 110
garlic and herbs (*Lea & Perrins*) 40
hickory (*Open Pit/Open Pit* Thick and Tangy) 50
hickory and brown sugar (*Hunt's*) 75
hickory or honey hickory (*Hunt's/Hunt's* Bold) 40
honey (*Heinz* Thick & Rich) 45
honey Dijon (*KC Masterpiece*) 50
honey mustard (*Hunt's*) 45
honey and spice (*Open Pit* Thick and Tangy) 45
hot and spicy or teriyaki (*Hunt's*) 45
onion (*Open Pit/Open Pit* Thick and Tangy) 50
Oriental, pork (*House of Tsang*) 90
sweet and sour (*Open Pit*) 45
Barley, pearled:
uncooked (*Arrowhead Mills*), ¼ cup 170
quick, uncooked (*Quaker* Scotch Quick), ⅓ cup 170
Barley flakes, rolled (*Arrowhead Mills*), ⅓ cup 110
Barley flour (*Arrowhead Mills*), ¼ cup 75
Basil, frozen (*Seabrook*), 1 tbsp., ¼ oz. 2
Bass, meat only:
freshwater, baked, broiled, or microwaved, 4 oz. 166
striped, baked, broiled, or microwaved, 4 oz. 141
Bean dip, 2 tbsp.:
(*Chi-Chi's* Fiesta) 35
(*Old Dutch*) 30
black bean (*Tostitos*) 30
hot (*Frito-Lay's*) 35
jalapeño (*Frito-Lay's*) 40
pinto, spicy (*Guiltless Gourmet*) 35
Bean dip mix, black or Mexican (*Knorr*), 1 tsp. 10
Bean dishes, mix (see also specific bean listings):
with bow tie pasta (*Bean Cuisine* Florentine), ½ cup* . . 199
with gemelli pasta (*Bean Cuisine* French Country),
½ cup* 214
Italian (*Knorr* Cup), 1 pkg. 230
red, with radiatore pasta (*Bean Cuisine* Barcelona),
½ cup* 170
with rice, see "Rice dishes"
Bean loaf, nine, frozen (*Natural Touch*), 1" slice 160

Bean salad, in jars:
deli style (*S&W*), ½ cup 80
marinated (*S&W*), ½ cup 70
Bean sauce, brown, spicy (*House of Tsang*), 1 tsp. 15
Beans, see "Baked beans," "Green beans" and other specific listings
Beans, mixed, canned (*Stokely* Chulent), ½ cup 110
Béarnaise sauce mix (*Knorr*), 1/10 pkg. 10
Beechnuts, dried, shelled, 1 oz. 164
Beef, choice meat only, trimmed to ¼" fat except as noted, 4 oz.:
brisket, whole, braised, lean with fat 437
brisket, whole, braised, lean only 274
chuck, arm pot roast, braised, lean with fat 395
chuck, arm pot roast, lean only 255
chuck, blade roast, braised, lean with fat 412
chuck, blade roast, lean only 298
flank steak, trimmed to 0" fat, braised, lean only 269
flank steak, trimmed to 0" fat, broiled, lean only 256
ground, raw, extra lean 265
ground, raw, lean 298
ground, raw, regular 351
ground, broiled medium, extra lean 290
ground, broiled medium, lean 308
ground, broiled medium, regular 328
porterhouse steak, broiled, lean with fat 346
porterhouse steak, broiled, lean only 247
rib, whole, roasted, lean with fat 426
rib, whole roasted, lean only 276
rib, large end (ribs 6–9), roasted, lean with fat 434
rib, large end (ribs 6–9), roasted, lean only 284
rib, small end (ribs 10–12), broiled, lean with fat 376
rib, small end (ribs 10–12), broiled, lean only 264
round, bottom, braised, lean with fat 322
round, bottom, braised, lean only 249
round, eye of, roasted, lean with fat 273
round, eye of, roasted, lean only 198
round, full cut, broiled, lean with fat 272
round, full cut, broiled, lean only 217

round, tip, roasted, lean with fat 280
round, tip, roasted, lean only 213
round, top, broiled, lean with fat 254
round, top, broiled, lean only 214
round, fried, lean with fat 314
round, fried, lean only 257
shank, crosscuts, braised, lean with fat 298
shank, crosscuts, braised, lean only 228
shortribs, braised, lean with fat 534
shortribs, braised, lean only 335
sirloin, top, broiled, lean with fat 305
sirloin, top, broiled, lean only 229
sirloin, top, fried, lean with fat 370
sirloin, top, fried, lean only 270
T-bone steak, broiled, lean with fat 338
T-bone steak, broiled, lean only 243
tenderloin, broiled, lean with fat 345
tenderloin, broiled, lean only 252
top loin, broiled, lean with fat 338
top loin, broiled, lean only 243

Beef, corned (see also "Beef hash" and "Beef lunch meat"):
brisket, cooked, 4 oz. 285
canned (*Hormel*), 2 oz. 120
canned, cubed (*Hormel*), ½ cup 130

Beef, dried (*Hormel,* 2½-oz. pkg.) 1 oz. 45

Beef dinner, frozen, 1 pkg.:
and broccoli (*Swanson*) 340
and broccoli (*Swanson Hungry Man*) 500
chicken fried steak (*Banquet*) 800
chicken fried steak with gravy (*Swanson*) 450
and gravy (*Swanson*) 310
and peppers, Cantonese (*Healthy Choice*) 270
pot roast, Yankee (*Swanson*) 260
pot roast, Yankee (*Swanson Hungry Man*) 400
roast beef sandwich, smothered (*Swanson*) 350
Salisbury steak (*Banquet*) 740
Salisbury steak (*Healthy Choice*) 320
Salisbury steak (*Swanson*) 420

Beef dinner *(cont.)*
Salisbury steak (*Swanson Hungry Man*) 590
sirloin, chopped, with gravy (*Swanson*) 310
sirloin tips (*Swanson Hungry Man*) 450
sirloin tips, with noodles (*Swanson*) 280
Stroganoff (*Healthy Choice*) 310
tips (*Healthy Choice* Traditional) 260
tips, with sauce (*Healthy Choice*) 290

Beef entree, canned:
chow mein (*La Choy* Bi-Pack), 1 cup 110
goulash (*Hormel*), 7.5-oz. can 230
hash, see "Beef hash"
pepper steak, Oriental (*La Choy* Bi-Pack), 1 cup 105
pepper steak with noodles, Oriental (*La Choy* Bi-Pack), 1 cup 160
pot roast (*Dinty Moore American Classics*), 10 oz. 210
roast, with gravy (*Hormel*), 2 oz. 60
roast, with mashed potato (*Dinty Moore American Classics*), 10 oz. 240
Salisbury steak (*Dinty Moore American Classics*), 10 oz. 310
stew (*Dinty Moore* Can/Cup), 7.5 oz. 190
stew (*Dinty Moore American Classics*), 10 oz. 260
stew (*Hunt's* Homestyle), 1 cup 155
stew, burger (*Dinty Moore* Hearty Cup), 7.5 oz. 240

Beef entree, frozen, 1 pkg., except as noted:
barbecue, mesquite (*Healthy Choice*) 310
broccoli Beijing (*Healthy Choice*) 330
chipped (*Banquet* Topper), 4 oz. 100
chipped, creamed (*Stouffer's*), 4.4 oz. 160
enchilada, see "Enchilada entree"
mesquite, with rice (*Lean Cuisine* Cafe Classics) 280
Oriental (*Lean Cuisine*) 250
Oriental (*Stouffer's Lunch Express*) 290
patty (*Swanson Fun Feast*) 470
patty, charbroiled, gravy and (*Morton*) 290
patty, gravy and (*Banquet*) 300
patty, mushroom gravy and (*Banquet*), 1 patty 180
patty, onion gravy and (*Banquet*), 1 patty 180
pepper steak (*The Budget Gourmet*) 290

pepper steak (*Stouffer's*) 330
pepper steak (*Weight Watchers*) 240
pepper steak, Oriental (*Healthy Choice*) 250
pie (*Banquet*) 330
pie (*Stouffer's*) 450
pie (*Swanson*) 400
pie (*Swanson Hungry Man*) 710
pot pie, Yankee (*Marie Callender's*) 690
pot roast, Yankee (*Marie Callender's*), 1 cup 640
pot roast, with potatoes (*Lean Cuisine*) 210
pot roast, with potatoes (*Stouffer's* Homestyle) 270
roast (*Healthy Choice* Hearty Handfuls), 6.1 oz. 310
Salisbury steak (*Banquet*) 310
Salisbury steak (*Healthy Choice*) 260
Salisbury steak (*Lean Cuisine*) 270
Salisbury steak (*Stouffer's* Homestyle) 370
Salisbury steak, gravy and (*Banquet*), 1 patty 200
Salisbury steak, gravy and (*Banquet* Toppers), 5 oz. . . . 220
Salisbury steak, gravy and (*Morton*) 210
Salisbury steak, gravy, mashed potato (*Swanson*) 310
Salisbury steak, grilled (*Weight Watchers*) 250
sandwich, see "Beef sandwich"
sirloin, peppercorn (*Lean Cuisine* Cafe Classics) 210
sirloin tips, and noodles (*Swanson*) 200
sliced (*Banquet* Country) 240
sliced, gravy and (*Banquet*), 2 slices 100
sliced, gravy and (*Banquet* Topper), 4 oz. 70
steak, chicken fried (*Banquet* Country) 400
steak, Philly (*Healthy Choice* Hearty Handfuls), 6.1 oz. . . 290
stew (*Banquet*), 1 cup 160
stir-fry (*Tyson* Kit), 1 cup 180
Stroganoff (*Stouffer's*) 390
tips, Français (*Healthy Choice*) 280
Beef gravy, hearty (*Pepperidge Farm*), 1/4 cup 25
Beef hash, canned:
(*Broadcast Morning Classics* Original), 1 cup 240
corned beef (*Dinty Moore* Cup), 7.5 oz. 200
corned beef (*Libby's*), 1 cup 490
corned beef or roast beef (*Mary Kitchen*), 1 cup 390

Beef hash *(cont.)*
roast beef (*Libby's*), 1 cup 460
sausage flavor (*Broadcast Morning Classics*), 1 cup . . . 240
Beef lunch meat (see also "Bologna" and "Pastrami"):
corned, brisket (*Boar's Head*), 2 oz. 80
corned, round (*Healthy Deli*), 2 oz. 80
roast (*Hormel*), 2 oz. 60
roast (*Hormel* Chuck), 2 oz. 110
roast (*Oscar Mayer Deli Thin*), 4 slices, 1.8 oz. 60
roast, seasoned or Italian style (*Healthy Deli*), 2 oz. 70
roast, round, eye, top, or pepper seasoned (*Boar's Head*), 2 oz. 90
Beef sandwich, frozen, 1 piece:
barbecue (*Hot Pockets*) 340
barbecue (*Hormel Quick Meal*) 360
and cheddar (*Hot Pockets*) 360
cheeseburger (*Hormel Quick Meal*) 400
cheeseburger, bacon (*Hormel Quick Meal*) 440
cheeseburger, chili (*Hormel Quick Meal*) 450
fajita (*Hot Pockets*) 360
hamburger (*Hormel Quick Meal*) 350
steak, biscuit (*Hormel Quick Meal*) 320
steak, and mushroom (*Mrs. Paterson's Aussie Pie*) 420
Beef spread, roast (*Underwood*), ¼ cup 130
Beef stew seasoning mix (*Lawry's* Spices & Seasonings), 2 tsp. 20
Beef Stroganoff sauce (*Lawry's*), 1 tbsp. 20
Beer:
regular, 12 fl. oz. 146
light, 12 fl. oz. 100
Beet:
fresh, boiled, sliced, drained, ½ cup 38
fresh, boiled, 2 medium, 2" diameter, approx. 3.5 oz. . . . 44
canned or in jars:
- whole (*Stokely*), 4.5 oz. 80
- whole, sliced, or julienne (*S&W*), ½ cup 30
- sliced (*Stokely*), ½ cup 40
- Harvard (*Stokely*), ⅓ cup 80

pickled, whole or sliced (*S&W*), 1 oz. 15
pickled, whole or sliced (*Stokely*), 1 oz. 25
Beet greens, fresh, boiled, drained, 1″ pieces, 1/2 cup . . . 20
Berry drink, 8 fl. oz.:
(*After the Fall* Oregon) 100
(*R. W. Knudson* Razzelberry) 130
citrus (*Five Alive*) 110
punch (*Minute Maid*) 120
Berry juice, 8 fl. oz.:
(*Apple & Eve Nothin' But Juice*) 120
(*Juicy Juice*) 130
(*Veryfine* Juice-Ups) 140
Biryani paste (*Patak's*), 2 tbsp. 160
Biscuit:
(*Arnold* Old Fashioned), 2 pieces 130
(*Awrey's* Country), 2 oz. 140
Biscuit, frozen, garlic and cheese (*Pepperidge Farm*),
1 piece 170
Biscuit, refrigerated:
(*Big Country* Buttermilk/Southern Style), 1 piece 100
(*Grands!* Homestyle or Flaky), 1 piece 190
(*Grands!* Buttermilk/Butter/Cinnamon Raisin/Southern),
1 piece 200
(*Hungry Jack/Hungry Jack Butter Tastin'*), 2 pieces 170
(*Hungry Jack Honey Tastin'/Hungry Jack Fluffy*), 2 pieces 180
(*Pillsbury* Butter/Buttermilk/Country), 3 pieces 150
Biscuit mix (see also "Baking mix"):
(*Arrowhead Mills*), 1/4 cup 120
(*Bisquick*), 1/3 cup 170
Black bean garlic sauce (*Lee Kum Kee*), 1 tbsp. 25
Black beans (see also "Refried beans"):
dried, boiled, 1/2 cup 113
canned (*Eden* Organic), 1/2 cup 100
canned (*S&W/Sun Vista*), 1/2 cup 70
canned, seasoned (*Allens/Trappey's*), 1/2 cup 120
Blackberry:
fresh, trimmed, 1/2 cup 37
canned (*Allens/Wolco*), 2/3 cup 60
canned, in heavy syrup, 1/2 cup 118

Blackberry ***(cont.)***
frozen, unsweetened, ½ cup 49
Black-eyed peas, ½ cup:
fresh, see "Cowpeas"
canned, fresh shell (*Stokely*) 110
canned, fresh shell, with jalapeño (*Homefolks*) 120
canned, fresh shell, with snaps (*Allens/East Texas Fair/ Homefolks*) 120
canned, dry (*Allens/East Texas Fair*) 110
Blintz, frozen:
apple (*Empire* Kosher), 2 pieces 220
blueberry or potato (*Empire* Kosher), 2 pieces 190
cheese or cherry (*Empire* Kosher), 2 pieces 200
Blood sausage, 1 oz. 107
Bloody Mary mixer (*V-8*), 11.5 fl. oz. 70
Blueberry:
fresh or frozen, unsweetened, ½ cup 40
canned in heavy syrup (*Lucky Leaf/Musselman's*), ½ cup 120
dried (*Sonoma*), ¼ cup 140
Bluefish, meat only, baked, broiled, or microwaved, 4 oz. 180
Bok choy, see "Cabbage"
Bologna (see also "Turkey bologna"):
(*Boar's Head*), 2 oz. 150
(*Healthy Deli* Regular/German 95% Fat Free), 2 oz. 70
(*John Morrell*), 2 oz. 180
beef or garlic (*Boar's Head*), 2 oz. 150
Bouillabaisse seasoning mix (*Knorr* Recipe), 1 tbsp. . . . 20
Bouillon (see also "Broth concentrate" and "Soup"):
all varieties (*Herb-Ox*), 1 cube 10
all varieties (*Herb-Ox* Instant), 1 tsp. or 1 pkt. 10
fish flavor (*Knorr*), ½ cube 10
vegetable, vegetarian (*Knorr*), ½ cube 15
Bourguignonne seasoning mix (*Knorr*), 1 tbsp. 35
Bow tie pasta mix, Italian cheese (*Lipton* Pasta & Sauce), ½ pkg. 230
Boysenberry:
fresh, trimmed, ½ cup 37
canned, in heavy syrup, ½ cup 113
frozen, unsweetened, ½ cup 33

Bran, see "Cereal," "Wheat bran," and specific bran listings
Bratwurst, cooked (*Jones Dairy Farm* Dinner), 1 link . . . 230
Braunschweiger:
chub (*Jones Dairy Farm* Original/Bacon/Onion), 2 oz. . . . 150
chunk (*Jones Dairy Farm* Original), 2 oz. 180
sliced (Oscar Mayer), 1 oz. slice 100
Brazil nuts, shelled, 1 oz., 6 large or 8 medium kernels 186
Bread, 1 slice, except as noted:
apple, honey wheat (*Brownberry*) 60
apple, walnut (*Pepperidge Farm*) 80
bran, honey (*Pepperidge Farm*) 90
bran, light (*August Bros./Brownberry Bakery* Country), 2 slices 80
bran, whole (*Brownberry* Natural) 60
brown, canned (*S&W*), ½ slice 90
buttermilk (*Arnold* Country) 100
cinnamon (*Brownberry*) 80
cranberry (*Arnold*) 70
date nut (*Thomas'*), 1 oz. 80
French (*Arnold Francisco*), 1 oz. 70
French (*Pepperidge Farm* Sliced), 1/9 loaf 120
golden, light (*Brownberry Bakery*), 2 slices 80
golden, swirl (*Pepperidge Farm* Vermont Maple) 90
grain and multigrain:
(*Brownberry* Hearth) 90
(*Roman Meal* Round Top/Sun) 70
5, sprouted (*Shiloh Farms/Shiloh Farms* No Salt) 90
7 (*Roman Meal*) 70
7, hearty (*Pepperidge Farm*) 100
7, light (*Pepperidge Farm*), 3 slices 140
7, light (*Roman Meal*), 2 slices 80
7, sprouted (*Shiloh Farms/Breads for Life*) 90
7, white (*Arnold/Brownberry Bran'nola*) 90
9 (*Pepperidge Farm*) 90
12 (*Arnold Bran'nola*) 90
12 (*Brownberry* Natural), 2 slices 110
12 (*Roman Meal*) 70
crunchy (*Pepperidge Farm*) 90

Bread, grain and multigrain *(cont.)*

nutty (*Arnold/Brownberry Bran'nola*) 90
with oat bran (*Roman Meal* Original) 70
sprouted (*Shiloh Farms* Sandwich) 80
whole (*Pepperidge Farm* 100%) 90
Italian (*Arnold Francisco*), 2 slices 110
Italian, brown and serve (*Pepperidge Farm*), 1/9 loaf 130
Italian, light (*Arnold/Brownberry Bakery*), 2 slices 80
Italian, stick, sliced (*Arnold Francisco* 1 lb.) 70
Italian, thick (*Brownberry Francisco*), 2 slices 110
kamut, sprout (*Shiloh Farms* Egyptian) 90
nut (*Brownberry* Natural Health) 70
oat (*Brownberry Bran'nola* Country) 90
oat (*Roman Meal*) 70
oat, crunchy, hearty (*Pepperidge Farm*) 100
oat bran, honey or honey nut (*Roman Meal*) 70
oat bran, light (*Roman Meal*), 2 slices 80
oatmeal (*Brownberry* Natural) 70
oatmeal (*Pepperidge Farm*) 80
oatmeal, light (*Arnold/Brownberry Bakery*), 2 slices 80
oatmeal, light (*Pepperidge Farm*), 3 slices 140
oatmeal, soft (*Brownberry*) 70
oatmeal, soft or thin (*Pepperidge Farm*) 60
orange raisin (*Brownberry*) 70
pita or pocket, 1 piece:
(*Arnold*), 2 oz. 140
(*Arnold*), 3 oz. 210
(*Pepperidge Farm*) 150
garlic (*Arnold*) 160
oat bran (*Thomas' Sahara*) 130
onion (*Arnold*) 150
salsa (*Thomas' Sahara*) 170
sourdough (*Thomas' Sahara*) 150
wheat (*Arnold* 4"), 1 oz. 70
wheat (*Arnold*), 2 oz. 140
wheat (*Arnold*), 3 oz. 200
white (*Arnold* 4"), 1 oz. 70
poppy seed, hazelnut (*Roman Meal*) 110
potato (*Arnold* Country) 100

potato, hearty (*Pepperidge Farm* Russet) 90
pumpernickel (*Arnold/Arnold Levy's/Arnold August Bros.* 1 lb.) 80
pumpernickel, dark (*Pepperidge Farm*) 80
pumpernickel or rye, party (*Pepperidge Farm*), 8 slices . . 110
pumpernickel, rye (*Brownberry* Natural) 70
raisin (*Arnold Sunmaid*) 70
raisin cinnamon (*Arnold/Brownberry*) 70
raisin cinnamon (*Pepperidge Farm*) 80
raisin walnut (*Brownberry*) 80
raisin whole wheat (*Shiloh Farms*), 2 slices 140
rye (*Arnold* Deli) 80
rye (*Brownberry* Hearth) 90
rye, Dijon (*Arnold* Real Jewish) 80
rye, Dijon, thin (*Pepperidge Farm*), 2 slices 100
rye, dill (*Arnold*) 80
rye, onion (*Arnold/August Bros.*) 80
rye, onion, seeded (*Arnold/August Bros.*) 90
rye, seeded or unseeded (*Arnold/August Bros.* 1 lb.) 80
rye, seeded or unseeded (*Arnold/Levy's* Real Jewish) 70
rye, seeded, unseeded, or dill (*Brownberry* Natural) 70
rye, seeded, unseeded, or onion (*Pepperidge Farm*) 80
rye, soft (*Arnold* Country) 70
rye, soft, light (*Arnold/Brownberry Bakery*), 2 slices 80
rye, soft, seeded or unseeded (*Arnold Bakery*) 80
rye, thin (*Arnold/August Bros./Arnold Levy's Melba*), 2 slices 90
rye, thin (*Brownberry*), 2 slices 100
rye and pump (*Arnold/August Bros.*) 90
sourdough (*Arnold/August Bros.*) 110
sourdough (*Arnold Francisco*) 90
sourdough, light (*Arnold*), 2 slices 80
sourdough, light (*Pepperidge Farm*), 3 slices 130
sourdough, thick (*Brownberry Francisco Int'l.*) 90
sourdough, whole grain (*Roman Meal*) 70
spelt (*Shiloh Farms*) 100
stick, sliced (*Arnold/August Bros.*), 2 slices 110
stick, sliced (*Brownberry Francisco Int'l.*) 100
toast, Texas (*Arnold/August Bros.*) 150

Bread *(cont.)*
Vienna, light (*Pepperidge Farm*), 3 slices 130
Vienna, thick (*Pepperidge Farm*) 70
wheat (*Arnold* Brick Oven 8 oz. or 16 oz.) 110
wheat (*Arnold* Brick Oven/*Brownberry* Natural) 80
wheat (*Arnold Sunny Valley*), 2 slices 100
wheat (*Arnold/Brownberry* Country/*Brownberry* Hearth) . . . 90
wheat (*Pepperidge Farm/Pepperidge Farm* Natural) 90
wheat (*Pepperidge Farm* Family) 70
wheat (*Roman Meal* Natural) 90
wheat (*Shiloh Farms* Homestyle), ½" slice, 2 oz. 160
wheat, cracked, thin (*Pepperidge Farm*) 70
wheat, dark or hearty (*Arnold Bran'nola/Brownberry Bran'nola*) 90
wheat, light (*Pepperidge Farm*), 3 slices 130
wheat, light or hearty light (*Roman Meal*), 2 slices 80
wheat, light, golden (*Arnold*), 2 slices 80
wheat, sesame, hearty (*Pepperidge Farm*) 100
wheat, soft (*Brownberry*) 80
wheat, soft (*Brownberry* 16 oz.), 2 slices 110
wheat, very thin (*Pepperidge Farm*), 3 slices 110
wheat, whole (*Arnold* 100% Stoneground 1 lb. 4 oz.) . . . 60
wheat, whole (*Roman Meal* 100%) 60
wheat, whole (*Shiloh Farms/Shiloh Farms* No Salt), 2 slices 140
wheat, whole, light (*Roman Meal* 100%), 2 slices 80
wheat, whole, soft or thin (*Pepperidge Farm*) 60
wheatberry, honey (*Arnold*) 70
wheatberry, honey (*Arnold Bran'nola*) 90
wheatberry, honey (*Roman Meal*) 70
wheatberry, honey, hearty (*Pepperidge Farm*) 100
wheatberry, honey light (*Roman Meal*), 2 slices 80
white (*Arnold* Brick Oven) 80
white (*Arnold* Brick Oven 1 lb.), 2 slices 130
white (*Arnold/Arnold Sunny Valley*), 2 slices 100
white (*Brownberry* Country) 90
white (*Brownberry* Natural), 2 slices 120
white, hearty (*Pepperidge Farm/Pepperidge Farm* Country) 90

white, light (*Arnold/Brownberry Bakery* Premium), 2 slices 80
white, light (*Roman Meal*), 2 slices 80
white, sandwich (*Pepperidge Farm*), 2 slices 130
white, sandwich (*Roman Meal*), 2 slices 110
white, soft (*Brownberry* 16 oz.), 2 slices 110
white, soft (*Brownberry/Arnold* Country) 80
white, thin (*Pepperidge Farm*) 80
white, very thin (*Pepperidge Farm*), 3 slices 110
white, toasting (*Pepperidge Farm*) 90

Bread, frozen, 1/6 loaf, except as noted:
cheddar, two (*Pepperidge Farm*) 210
garlic or garlic Parmesan (*Pepperidge Farm*) 160
garlic, mozzarella (*Pepperidge Farm*) 200
garlic, sourdough (*Pepperidge Farm*) 180
Monterey jack or jalapeño cheese (*Pepperidge Farm*) . . . 200
white, dough (*Rich's*), 2.2 oz. 150

Bread, refrigerated:
(*Pillsbury Pipin' Hot*), 1/6 loaf 110
corn bread twists (*Pillsbury*), 1 twist 130
French (*Pillsbury*), 1/5 loaf 150

Bread, stuffed, refrigerated:
broccoli and cheese (*Stuffed Breads*), 6 oz. 450
pepperoni and cheese (*Stuffed Breads*), 6 oz. 610

Bread crumbs:
(*Contadina*), 1/3 cup 100
all varieties (*Devonsheer/Old London*), 1/4 cup or 1 oz. . . 100

Bread mix (see also "Bread mix, sweet"):
beer (*Buckeye*), 1/14 pkg. 130
beer, whole wheat (*Buckeye*), 1/14 pkg. 120
cheddar cheese or Italian herb (*Dromedary*), 1/9 pkg. . . . 140
corn bread (*Arrowhead Mills*), 1/4 cup 120
corn bread (*Aunt Jemima* Easy Mix), 1/3 cup 150
corn bread (*Buckeye*), 1/16 pkg. 130
corn bread (*Dromedary*), 1/10 pkg. 140
kamut (*Arrowhead Mills*), 1/3 cup 140
multigrain or rye (*Arrowhead Mills*), 1/3 cup 160
oatmeal, honey (*Dromedary*), 1/9 pkg. 150
sourdough (*Buckeye*), 1/14 pkg. 130

Bread mix *(cont.)*
sourdough or stoneground wheat (*Dromedary*), 1/9 pkg. 140
spelt (*Arrowhead Mills*), 1/3 cup 150
wheat, cracked (*Pillsbury* Bread Machine), 1/2 loaf* 130
wheat, whole (*Arrowhead Mills*), 1/3 cup 150
white (*Arrowhead Mills*), 1/3 cup 150
white, country (*Dromedary*), 1/9 pkg. 140
white, crusty (*Pillsbury* Bread Machine), 1/12 loaf* 130
Bread mix, sweet:
apple cinnamon (*Dromedary*), 1/9 pkg. 140
apple cinnamon (*Pillsbury*), 1/2 loaf* 180
banana or pumpkin (*Pillsbury*), 1/12 pkg.* 170
blueberry or cranberry (*Pillsbury*), 1/12 loaf* 180
carrot (*Pillsbury*), 1/12 pkg.* 140
date (*Pillsbury*), 1/12 pkg.* 180
date nut (*Dromedary*), 1/12 pkg. 180
gingerbread (*Dromedary*), 1/6 pkg. 260
gingerbread (*Pillsbury* Bread Machine), 1/8 loaf* 220
nut (*Pillsbury*), 1/12 pkg.* 190
Bread snacks:
cinnamon raisin swirl (*Pepperidge Farm* Bread Crisps),
1 oz. 130
garlic butter swirl (*Pepperidge Farm* Bread Crisps), 1 oz. 140
sticks, pretzel (*Pepperidge Farm*), 9 sticks 130
sticks, pumpernickel or sesame (*Pepperidge Farm*),
9 sticks 150
sticks, three cheese (*Pepperidge Farm*), 9 sticks 140
Bread stick:
(*Pepperidge Farm* Brown and Serve), 1 stick 150
(*Pillsbury*), 1 stick 110
(*Stella D'Oro*), 1 stick 40
(*Stella D'Oro* Fat Free Original), 5 sticks 60
(*Stella D'Oro* Fat Free Traditional), 2 sticks 70
(*Stella D'Oro* No Sodium), 1 stick 45
cheddar, thin (*Pepperidge Farm*), 7 sticks 70
cheese (*Handi-Snacks*), 1 stick 130
cheese, three (*Pepperidge Farm*), 9 sticks 140
garlic (*Stella D'Oro* Fat Free Deli), 5 sticks 60
garlic (*Stella D'Oro* Fat Free Traditional), 2 sticks 70

garlic, onion, or wheat (*Stella D'Oro*), 1 stick 40
onion, thin (*Pepperidge Farm*), 7 sticks 70
pretzel (*Pepperidge Farm*), 9 sticks 130
pumpernickel or sesame (*Pepperidge Farm*), 9 sticks . . . 150
sesame (*Stella D'Oro/Stella D'Oro* No Sodium), 1 stick . . . 50
sesame (*Stella D'Oro* Low Fat), 2 pieces 70
sesame thin (*Pepperidge Farm*), 7 sticks 60
Broad beans, fresh, boiled, drained, 4 oz. 64
Broad beans, mature:
dry (*Frieda's* Fava Beans), 1 oz. 15
dry, boiled, ½ cup 93
canned, with liquid (*Progresso* Fava Beans), ½ cup 110
Broccoli:
fresh, raw (*Dole*), 1 medium stalk 40
fresh, raw, florets (*Dole*), 3 oz. 25
boiled, drained, 1 spear, 6.3 oz. 51
boiled, drained, chopped, ½ cup 22
frozen, chopped (*Seabrook*), ¾ cup, 3 oz. 25
frozen, cuts (*Green Giant*), 1 cup 25
frozen, florets (*Green Giant*), 1⅓ cup 25
frozen, spears (*Green Giant*), 3 oz. 25
frozen, spears, in butter sauce (*Green Giant*), 4 oz. 50
frozen, in cheese sauce (*Green Giant*), ⅔ cup 70
Broccoli combinations, frozen:
cauliflower, carrots (*Green Giant Harvest Fresh*), 1 cup . . . 30
cauliflower, carrots, and cheese sauce (*Green Giant*),
⅔ cup 80
cauliflower, carrots, corn, peas, and butter sauce (*Green Giant*), ¾ cup 60
stir-fry (*Bird's Eye*), 1 cup 30
stir-fry (*Green Giant Create-A-Meal*), 2⅓ cup 120
Broccoli and cheddar, frozen:
pocket (*Ken & Robert's Veggie Pockets*), 1 piece 250
pot pie (*Amy's*), 7.5 oz. 430
Broth, see "Soup"
Broth concentrate (see also "Bouillon"):
beef or vegetable flavor (*Knorr*), 2 tsp. or 1 cup* 15
chicken flavor (*Knorr*), 2 tsp. or 1 cup* 5

Brown gravy, 1/4 cup:
with onions (*Franco-American*) 25
savory (*Heinz*) 25
mix* (*Durkee/French's*) 10
mix* (*Loma Linda Gravy Quik*) 20
mix*, herb (*Durkee/French's*) 15
Brown gravy sauce (*La Choy*), 1/4 cup 275
Brownie, 1 piece, except as noted:
chocolate (*Awrey's* Decadent), 1.9 oz. 230
chocolate, Bavarian (*Awrey's*), 2.1 oz. 250
chocolate, peanut (*Awrey's* Sensation) 1.9 oz. 230
fudge (*Little Debbie*), 2.5 oz. 310
fudge (*Awrey's*), 1.8 oz. 200
fudge nut (*Awrey's*) 1.6 oz. 190
fudge walnut (*Tastykake*) 3 oz. 360
mini (*Hostess Bites*) 5 pieces 260
mini, walnut (*Hostess Bites*) 5 pieces 270
Brownie, refrigerated, fudge (*Pillsbury*), 1/20 pkg. 160
Brownie mix:
(*Arrowhead Mills*), 1 piece* 110
(*Arrowhead Mills* Fat Free/Wheat Free), 1 piece* 120
cookies 'n creme (*Betty Crocker*), 1/18 pkg. 140
dark chocolate (*Betty Crocker*), 1/18 pkg. 130
fudge or walnut (*Betty Crocker*), 1/18 pkg. 140
Browning sauce (*Gravy Master*), 1/4 tsp. 10
Brussels sprouts:
fresh, boiled, drained, 1 sprout, .7 oz. 8
frozen (*Stilwell*), 6 sprouts, 3 oz. 35
frozen, baby, butter sauce (*Green Giant*), 2/3 cup 60
Buckwheat, whole grain, 1 cup 584
Buckwheat flour (*Arrowhead Mills*), 1/4 cup 100
Buckwheat groats:
brown (*Arrowhead Mills*), 1/4 cup 140
roasted, dry, 1 oz. 98
roasted, cooked, 1 cup 182
Bulgur (see also "Tabouli"):
dry (*Arrowhead Mills*), 1/4 cup 150
cooked, 1 cup 152
Bulgur pilaf mix (*Casbah*), 1 oz. 100

Bun, see "Roll"
Bun, honey (see also "Danish" and "Roll, sweet"):
(*Grandma's*), 1 bun 410
(*Little Debbie*), 3 oz. 380
(*Morton*), 2.3 oz. 290
(*Morton* Mini), 1.3 oz. 160
frozen (*Rich's*), 1 bun 240
glazed (*Hostess*), 2.7 oz. 320
iced (*Hostess*), 3.4 oz. 390
Burbot, meat only, baked, broiled, or microwaved, 4 oz. 130
Burdock root, boiled, drained, 1″ pieces, ½ cup 55
Burger, vegetarian, see " 'Hamburger,' vegetarian"
Burger King, 1 serving:
breakfast:
biscuit with bacon, egg, cheese 510
biscuit with sausage 590
Croissan'wich with sausage, egg, cheese 600
French toast sticks 500
hash browns 220
burgers, chicken, and sandwiches:
BK Big Fish 700
BK Broiler chicken 550
cheeseburger 380
cheeseburger, double 600
cheeseburger, double with bacon 640
chicken sandwich 710
Chicken Tenders, 6 pieces 230
Double Whopper 870
Double Whopper with cheese 960
hamburger 330
Whopper 640
Whopper with cheese 730
Whopper Jr. 420
Whopper Jr. with cheese 460
french fries, medium 370
onion rings 310
salad, broiled chicken, without dressing 200
salad, garden, without dressing 100
salad, side, without dressing 60

Burger King (cont.)
salad dressings, 1.2 oz.:
bleu cheese 160
French 140
Italian, light 15
ranch 180
Thousand Island 140
sauces, 1 oz., except as noted:
A.M. Express dip 80
barbecue dipping 35
Bull's Eye, .5 oz. 20
honey dipping 90
ranch dipping 170
sweet and sour dipping 45
shakes, medium:
chocolate 320
chocolate with syrup 440
strawberry with syrup 420
vanilla 300
Dutch apple pie 300

Burrito, frozen (see also "Burrito, breakfast" and "Burrito dinner"):
bean, black (*Amy's*), 6 oz. 320
bean and cheese (*Tina's*), 5 oz. 340
bean and rice (*Amy's*), 6 oz. 250
bean and rice with cheese (*Amy's*), 6 oz. 280
beef (*Hormel QuickMeal*), 4 oz. 300
beef, spicy (*Tina's* Red Hot), 5 oz. 370
beef, nacho (*Patio Britos*), 6 oz. 410
beef and bean (*Patio Britos*), 6 oz. 420
beef steak and bean (*Don Miguel*), 7 oz. 370
cheese (*Hormel Quick Meal*), 4 oz. 250
cheese, nacho (*Patio Britos*), 6 oz. 360
chicken (*Don Miguel*), 7 oz. 360
chicken and cheese, spicy (*Patio Britos*), 6 oz. 400
chicken con queso (*Healthy Choice*), 5.4 oz. 280
chili, red (*Hormel Quick Meal*), 4 oz. 280

Burrito, breakfast, frozen, 1 pkg.:
black bean (*Amy's*) 230

egg, scrambled (*Swanson Great Starts* Original) 200
egg and bacon (*Swanson Great Starts*) 250
ham and cheese (*Swanson Great Starts*) 210
hot and spicy (*Swanson Great Starts*) 220
pizza, with cheese and pepperoni (*Swanson Great Starts*) 240
sausage (*Swanson Great Starts*) 240

Burrito dinner, frozen:
beef (*Chi-Chi's* Burro), 15 oz. 570
chicken (*Chi-Chi's* Burro Chix), 15 oz. 530

Burrito sauce (*Hunt's Manwich*), ¼ cup 25

Burrito seasoning mix (*Lawry's*), 1 tbsp. 35

Butter, salted or unsalted:
regular, 1 tbsp. 100
whipped, 1 tbsp. 67

Butter beans, see "Lima beans"

Butterfish, meat only, baked, broiled, or microwaved, 4 oz. 212

Buttermilk, see "Milk"

Butternut, shelled, 1 oz. 174

Butternut squash, boiled, drained, mashed, ½ cup 47

Butterscotch chips, baking (*Nestlé* Morsels), 1 tbsp. 80

Butterscotch topping:
(*Kraft*), 2 tbsp. 130
(*Smucker's* Sundae), 2 tbsp. 110

Butterscotch-caramel topping (*Smucker's*), 2 tbsp. 130

C

FOOD AND MEASURE	CALORIES
Cabbage, 1/2 cup, except as noted:	
fresh, raw, shredded	9
fresh, boiled, drained, shredded	17
bok choy, fresh, boiled, drained, shredded	10
napa, fresh, raw, shredded (*Dole*), 3 oz.	6
pe-tsai, fresh, boiled, drained, shredded	8
red or savoy, fresh, raw, shredded	10
red or savoy, fresh, boiled, drained, shredded	18
red, in jars, sweet and sour (*S&W*), 2 tbsp.	15
Cabbage, stuffed, with potato, frozen (*Lean Cuisine*), 9 1/2 oz.	220
Cactus leaves (*Frieda's*), 3/4 cup, 3 oz.	20
Cake:	
angel food ring (*Hostess*), 1/6 cake	150
banana, (*Awrey's* Sheet), 1/24 cake	350
banana chocolate chip (*Awrey's* Marquise), 1/16 cake	310
Black Forest torte (*Awrey's*), 1/12 cake	350
Boston creme (*Awrey's*), 1/16 cake	190
carrot, cream cheese iced, 2 layer (*Awrey's*), 1/16 cake	390
cherries cordial (*Awrey's* Marquise), 1/16 cake	240
chocolate, double (*Awrey's*), 1/12 cake	340
chocolate, German, 3 layer (*Awrey's*), 1/16 cake	360
chocolate, peanut fantasy (*Awrey's* Marquise), 1/16 cake	330
chocolate, tropical (*Awrey's* Marquise), 1/16 cake	230
chocolate, white iced, 2 layer (*Awrey's*), 1/16 cake	270
coconut buttercream, 3 layer (*Awrey's*), 1/16 cake	360
coffee (*Awrey's* Long John), 1/12 cake	190
espresso, French (*Awrey's* Marquise), 1/16 cake	320
fruit cake (*Hostess* 2 lb.), 1/6 cake	490
lemon, 3 layer (*Awrey's*), 1/16 cake	320
Neapolitan (*Awrey's*), 1/12 cake	360
orange, 3 layer (*Awrey's*), 1/16 cake	330
peach, Georgia (*Awrey's* Marquise), 1/16 cake	260

pound (*Hostess*), 1/5 cake 350
pound, golden (*Awrey's*), 1/6 cake 250
raspberry and creme (*Awrey's* Marquise), 1/16 cake 260
raspberry nut (*Awrey's* Marquise), 1/16 cake 310
sponge, uniced (*Awrey's*), 1/24 cake 190
strawberry supreme (*Awrey's* Marquise), 1/16 cake 240
strawberry supreme torte (*Awrey's*), 1/12 cake 270
yellow, lemon iced, 2 layer (*Awrey's*), 1/16 cake 290
yellow, white iced (*Awrey's* Sheet), 1/24 cake 360

Cake, frozen:

Boston creme (*Mrs. Smith's*), 1/8 cake 170
carrot (*Pepperidge Farm* Deluxe), 1/8 cake 310
cheesecake, French strawberry (*Sara Lee*), 1/6 cake 320
cheesecake, strawberry (*Amy's*), 4 oz. 290
chocolate, double, layer (*Sara Lee*), 1/6 cake 260
chocolate, fudge (*Amy's*), 3.25 oz. 320
coconut or chocolate fudge layer (*Pepperidge Farm*), 1/6 cake 300
coffee cake (*Sara Lee*), 1/8 cake 220
devil's food, golden, or vanilla layer (*Pepperidge Farm*), 1/6 cake 290
pound, butter (*Pepperidge Farm*), 1/5 cake 290

Cake, mix*, 1/12 cake or pkg., except as noted:

angel food (*Betty Crocker*) 150
angel food (*Pillsbury Moist Supreme*) 140
banana or carrot (*Pillsbury Plus/Moist Supreme*) 260
butter recipe (*Pillsbury Plus/Moist Supreme*) 260
butter recipe chocolate (*Pillsbury Moist Supreme*) 260
cheesecake, (*Jell-O* Real) 1/6 cake 350
cheesecake, cherry (*Jell-O*) 1/6 cake 330
chocolate (*Pillsbury Moist Supreme*) 250
chocolate chip (*Pillsbury Plus/Moist Supreme*) 240
chocolate, dark (*Pillsbury Plus/Moist Supreme*) 250
chocolate, German (*Pillsbury Plus/Moist Supreme*) 250
cinnamon streusel (*Pillsbury Streusel Swirl*), 1/16 cake . . 260
confetti (*Pillsbury Plus/Moist Supreme Funfetti*) 240
devil's food (*Pillsbury Plus/Moist Supreme*) 270
fudge swirl (*Pillsbury Moist Supreme*) 250
gingerbread, see "Bread mix, sweet"

Cake, mix *(cont.)*

lemon (*Pillsbury Moist Supreme*), 1/10 cake 300
strawberry (*Pillsbury Plus*) 260
vanilla, French (*Pillsbury Moist Supreme*), 1/10 cake 300
vanilla, sunshine (*Pillsbury Plus/Moist Supreme*) 260
white, (*Pillsbury Plus/Moist Supreme*), 1/10 cake 280
white 'n fudge swirl (*Pillsbury Plus/Moist Supreme*) . . . 250
yellow (*Pillsbury Moist Supreme*) 240

Cake, snack:

all varieties (*Health Valley* Healthy Tarts Fat Free), 1 cake 150
almond, cinnamon, or coconut twirl (*Aunt Fanny's*), 1 oz. 110
apple or apricot bar (*Health Valley* Fat Free) 140
banana (*Little Debbie* Twins), 2.2 oz. 250
banana or chocolate (*Suzy Q's*), 2 oz. 220
banana (*Twinkies*), 2 cakes 300
Boston creme (*Drake's*), 1.5 oz. 170
brownie bar, fudge filled (*Health Valley* Fat Free), 1 cake 110
cheesecake (*Boar's Head* New York), 4 oz. 380
chocolate (*Ding Dongs*), 1.3 oz. 160
chocolate (*Ho-Hos*), 1 oz. 130
chocolate (*Yodels*), 2 cakes, 2.2 oz. 280
chocolate chip (*Little Debbie*), 2.2 oz. 280
coconut covered (*Sno Balls*), 1.6 oz. 160
coffee cake (*Drake's*), 1.1 oz. 130
crumb (*Hostess*), 2 cakes 210
cupcake, buttercreme, iced (*Tastykake*), 2 cakes 250
cupcake, chocolate (*Hostess*), 1.6 oz. 170
cupcake, chocolate creme, iced (*Tastykake*), 2 cakes . . . 250
cupcake, mini, all varieties (*Tastykake*), 2 cakes 110
cupcake, orange (*Hostess*), 1.5 oz. 160
date or raisin bar (*Health Valley* Fat Free), 1 cake 140
devil's food (*Little Debbie Devil Cremes*), 3.2 oz. 370
dunking stick (*Little Debbie*), 2 oz. 250
fruit loaf (*Hostess*), 3.8 oz. 350
fudge frosted (*Little Debbie*), 2.2 oz. 270
golden, creme-filled (*Twinkies*), 1.4 oz. 140
pecan twirl (*Aunt Fanny's*), 1 oz. 100
pound (*Tastykake*), 3 oz. 320
strawberry shortcake (*Little Debbie*), 1 cake 290

Swiss roll (*Little Debbie*), 2.7 oz. 320
vanilla (*Little Debbie*), 3 oz. 380
vanilla fingers (*Aunt Fanny's*), 2 cakes, 3 oz. 290
yellow (*Hostess* Baseball), 1.7 oz. 160
zebra cake (*Little Debbie*), 3 oz. 380

Calzone, refrigerated:
cheese (*Stefano's*), 6-oz. piece 510
pepperoni (*Stefano's*), 6-oz. piece 520
spinach (*Stefano's*), 6-oz. piece 440

Candy:
(*Baby Ruth*), 2.1-oz. bar 280
(*Bar None*), 1.65-oz. bar 250
all flavors (*Pearson's Nips*), 2 pieces 60
buttercrunch, with almond (*Almond Roca*), 4 pieces . . . 280
(*Butterfinger*), 2.1-oz. bar 280
butterscotch (*Brach's Disks*), 3 pieces 70
caramel, chocolate coated (*Rolo*), 1.9 oz. 260
caramel, with cookies (*Twix*), 1-oz. piece 140
cherry, chocolate covered (*Perugina*), 1.21 oz. 160
chocolate, with hazelnuts (*Ferraro Rocher*), 3 pieces . . . 220
chocolate, candy coated, plain (*M&M's*), 1½ oz. 200
chocolate, candy coated, with almonds, peanuts, or
peanut butter (*M&M's*), 1½ oz. 220
chocolate, dark (*Ghirardelli*), 1¼-oz. bar 180
chocolate, dark (*Hershey's Special Dark*), 1.45-oz. bar . . 230
chocolate, dark, with almonds (*Ghirardelli*), 1½-oz. bar . . 220
chocolate, milk (*Ghirardelli*), 1¼-oz. bar 190
chocolate, milk (*Hershey's Hugs/Hershey's Kisses*),
8 pieces 210
chocolate, milk, with almonds (*Ghirardelli*), 1¼-oz. bar . . 170
chocolate, milk, with caramel (*Caramello*), 1.6-oz. bar . . 220
chocolate, milk, cookies and cream (*Ghirardelli*), 1.3 oz. 190
chocolate, milk, with crisps (*Ghirardelli*), 1¼-oz. bar . . . 180
chocolate, milk, with fruit and nuts (*Chunky*), 1.4-oz. bar 200
chocolate, milk, with hazelnuts (*Mon Cheri*), 3 pieces . . . 260
chocolate, milk, with peanuts (*Mr. Goodbar*), 1¾-oz. bar 270
chocolate, milk, thins (*Lindt* Swiss), 15 pieces, 1½ oz. . . 230
chocolate, with toffee (*Ghirardelli*), 4 pieces, 1½ oz. . . . 220

Candy *(cont.)*

chocolate, white, raspberry cream (*Ghirardelli*), 4 pieces, ⅓ oz. 200
coconut, chocolate coated (*Mounds*), 1.9-oz. bar 250
coconut, chocolate coated, with almonds (*Almond Joy*), 1.76-oz. bar 240
fruit flavor, gummed (*Gummi Savers*), 1½ oz. 130
gum, chewing (*Beech-Nut*), 1 piece 10
gum, bubble (*Bubble Yum*), 1 piece 25
hard, all flavors (*Brach's Sparklers*), 3 pieces, .6 oz. 70
hard, all flavors except mints (*Lifesavers*), 2 pieces 20
hard, chocolate dipped (*Bogdon's* Reception Sticks), 1 piece 16
honey (*Bit-O-Honey*), 1.7-oz. bar 200
jelled (*Jujubes/Jujyfruits*), 1.4 oz. 160
jelled, spearmint leaves (*Brach's*), 5 pieces 130
licorice, regular or strawberry (*Twizzlers*), 4 pieces, 1½ oz. 140
licorice, candy coated (*Good & Plenty*), 1.4 oz. 130
lollipop, all flavors, (*Life Savers*), 1 pop, .4 oz. 40
malted milk balls (*Whoppers*), 1.4 oz. 190
(*Mars* Bar), 1.76 oz. 240
(*Milky Way*), 2.15 oz. 280
mint, all flavors except *Cryst-O-Mint* (*Lifesavers*), 3 pieces 20
mint (*Life Savers Cryst-O-Mint*), 2 pieces 20
mint, butter (*Kraft*), 7 pieces 60
mint, chocolate coated (*After Eight*), 5 pieces 190
(*Nestlé Turtles*), 2 pieces 160
nonpareils (*Ghirardelli*), 1.4 oz. 190
nougat (*Brach's*), 4 pieces 170
(*Pay Day*), 1.85-oz. bar 250
peanut (*Planters*), 1.6-oz. bar 230
peanut brittle (*Kraft*), 1.3 oz. 170
peanut butter, chocolate (*5th Avenue*), 2-oz. bar 280
peanut butter cup (*Reese's*), 1½-oz. pkg. 250
raisins, chocolate coated (*Raisinets*), 1.58 oz. 200
(*Snickers*), 2.07-oz. bar 280
(*3 Musketeers*), 2.13-oz. bar 260

toffee (*Brach's* Treasures), 3 pieces 80
toffee bar (*Skor*), 1.4 oz. 220
(*Tootsie Roll* Midges), 6 pieces, 1.4 oz. 160
wafer, chocolate coated (*Kit Kat*), 1½-oz. bar 220
(*Whatchamacallit*), 1.7-oz. bar 250
Cane syrup, 1 tbsp. 52
Cannellini beans, see "Kidney beans"
Cannelloni dinner, frozen (*Amy's*), 10 oz. 260
Cannelloni entree, cheese, frozen (*Lean Cuisine*), 9⅛ oz. 240
Cantaloupe, fresh:
½ of 5″-diameter melon 94
pulp, cubed, ½ cup 29
Cantaloupe drink (*Snapple* Cocktail), 8 fl. oz. 130
Capers:
(*Crosse and Blackwell*), 1 tbsp. 5
with pimientos (*Goya*), ¼ cup 25
Cappuccino, iced:
(*Jamaican Gold*), 11 fl. oz. 145
coffee (*Maxwell House*), 8 fl. oz. 130
mocha or vanilla (*Maxwell House*), 8 fl. oz. 140
Cappuccino mix, see "Coffee, flavored, mix"
Cappuccino bar, frozen (*Frozfruit*), 1 bar 140
Carambola:
fresh (*Frieda's*), 3.5 oz. 35
dried (*Frieda's*), 1 oz. 77
dried (*Sonoma*), 1.4 oz., 7–9 pieces 140
Caramel dip (*Marie's*), 2 tbsp. 150
Caramel topping, syrup (*Smucker's* Sundae), 2 tbsp. . . 110
Carbonara sauce mix (*Knorr*), 2 tbsp. 70
Carissa, 1 medium, .8 oz. 12
Carl's Jr., 1 serving:
breakfast dishes:
    bacon, 2 strips 40
    breakfast burrito 430
    breakfast quesadilla 300
    English muffin, with margarine 230
    French toast dips, without syrup 410
    jelly, grape or strawberry 35
    sausage, 1 patty 200

Carl's Jr.*, breakfast dishes *(cont.)

scrambled eggs 160
Sunrise Sandwich 370
table syrup, 1 oz. 90
chicken stars, 6 pieces 230
sauces:
barbecue 50
honey 90
mustard 45
salsa 10
sweet n' sour 50
sandwiches:
Big Burger 470
Carl's Catch Fish Sandwich 560
chicken bacon Swiss 670
chicken, barbecued 310
chicken club 550
chicken, ranch 580
chicken, Santa Fe 530
double cheeseburger, ⅓ lb. 660
Double Western Bacon Cheeseburger 970
Famous Big Star hamburger 610
hamburger 200
Hot & Crispy sandwich 400
Super Star hamburger 820
Western Bacon Cheeseburger 870
"Great Stuff" potatoes:
bacon and cheese 630
broccoli and cheese 530
plain 290
sour cream and chive 430
Entree Salads-To-Go:
chicken 260
garden 50
salad dressing, 2 oz.:
blue cheese 310
French, fat free 70
house 220
Italian, fat free 15

Thousand Island 250
side dishes:
CrissCut Fries, large 550
regular fries 370
hash brown nuggets 270
onion rings 520
zucchini 380
shakes, small:
chocolate 390
strawberry 400
vanilla 330
desserts and bakery products:
blueberry muffin 340
bran muffin 370
cheese danish 400
cheesecake, strawberry swirl 300
chocolate cake 300
chocolate chip cookie 370
cinnamon roll 420
Carob drink mix, powder, 3 tsp. 45
Carp, meat only, baked, broiled, or microwaved, 4 oz. . . 184
Carrot:
fresh, raw, whole, 7½" long, 2.8 oz. 31
fresh, raw, shredded or mini, peeled (*Dole*), 3 oz. 50
fresh, boiled, drained, sliced, ½ cup 35
canned, all varieties (*S&W*), ½ cup 25
canned, whole or sliced (*Stokely*), 4.5 oz. 30
frozen, baby, cut (*Green Giant Harvest Fresh*), ⅔ cup . . . 20
Casaba, fresh:
1/10 of 7¾" melon 43
pulp, cubed, ½ cup 23
Cashew:
dry-roasted or oil-roasted, 1 oz. or 18 medium 163
honey-roasted (*Planters*), 1 oz. 150
oil-roasted (*Planters* Fancy), 1 oz. 170
Cashew butter (*Roaster Fresh*), 1 oz. 165
Cassava (see also "Yuca"), fresh, 1 oz. 34
Catfish, channel, 4 oz.:
farmed, meat only, baked, broiled, or microwaved 172

wild, meat only, baked, broiled, or microwaved 119
Catfish, frozen, fillets (*Delta Pride*), 4 oz. 90
Catjang, boiled, ½ cup 100
Cauliflower:
fresh, raw, florets (*Dole*), 3 oz. 20
fresh, boiled, drained, 1″ pieces, ½ cup 14
fresh, green, raw, (*Dole*), ⅕ head 35
fresh, green, boiled, drained, 1″ pieces, ½ cup 20
frozen, florets (*Green Giant*), 1 cup 25
frozen, in cheese sauce (*Green Giant*), ½ cup 60
Cauliflower, pickled, sweet, in jars (*Vlasic*), 1 oz. 35
Caviar, 1 tbsp.:
black or red 40
carp roe (*Krinos* Tarama) 20
lumpfish, black or red (*Romanoff*) 15
salmon, red (*Romanoff*) 35
whitefish, black (*Romanoff*) 25
Caviar spread (*Krinos* Taramasalata), 1 tbsp. 90
Celeriac, fresh, boiled, drained, 4 oz. 28
Celery, fresh:
raw, 7½″-stalk, 1.6 oz. 6
raw, diced, ½ cup 10
Celtus, raw, trimmed, 1 oz. 6
Cereal, ready-to-eat:
bran (*Nabisco 100% Bran*), ⅓ cup 80
bran, raisin (*New Morning* Multi-Bran), 1 cup 90
bran, raisin (*Post*), 1 cup 190
bran flakes (*New Morning* Multi-Bran), 1 cup 110
bran flakes (*Post*), ⅔ cup 90
corn, almond raisin (*New Morning Crunchy*), ¾ cup . . . 110
corn, flakes (*Kellogg's Corn Flakes*), 1 cup 110
corn, flakes (*New Morning*), 1 cup 120
corn and rice (*Kellogg's Crispix*), 1 cup 110
granola (*C.W. Post* Hearty), ⅔ cup 280
granola (*New Morning Oatiola*), ¾ cup 200
granola, raisin (*Heartland*), ½ cup 290
mixed grain (*Fruit & Fibre*), 1 cup 210
mixed grain (*Grape-Nuts*), ½ cup 200
mixed grain, flakes (*Grape-Nuts* Flakes), ¾ cup 100

mixed grain, flakes (*Product 19*), 1 cup 110
oat (*Alpha-Bits*), 1 cup 130
oat (*Honey Bunches of Oats*), 3/4 cup 120
oat (*New Morning Oatios* Original), 1 cup 120
oat (*Toasty O's*), 1 cup 110
oat, with almonds (*Honey Bunches of Oats*), 3/4 cup . . . 130
oat, apple cinnamon (*New Morning Oatios*), 1 cup 90
oat, honey almond (*New Morning Oatios*), 1 cup 100
oat, honey graham (*Quaker Oh!s*), 3/4 cup 110
oat bran (*New Morning Ultimate Oat Bran*), 1 cup 110
rice (*Special K*), 1 cup 110
rice, crispy (*Malt-O-Meal), 1 cup* 110
rice, puffed (*Malt-O-Meal), 1 cup* 60
rice and corn, almond raisin (*Nutri-Grain*), 1 1/4 cups . . . 200
rice and rye (*Kellogg's Apple Raisin Crisp*), 1 cup 180
wheat (*Nabisco Frosted Wheat Bites*), 1 cup 190
wheat (*Nutri-Grain* Golden), 3/4 cup 100
wheat, puffed (*Malt-O-Meal), 1 cup* 50
wheat, with raisins (*Nutri-Grain* Golden), 1 1/4 cups 180
wheat, shredded (*Nabisco*), 2 biscuits 160
wheat, shredded (*Nabisco Spoon Size*), 1 cup 170
Cereal, cooking, uncooked, 1 pkt., except as noted:
farina, see "wheat," below
mixed grain (*Roman Meal*) 130
mixed grain (*Roman Meal* Instant) 100
oat flakes, raisin and spice (*H-O* Instant) 150
oatmeal (*H-O* Instant), 1/2 cup 150
oatmeal (*Quaker* Instant) 130
oats (*H-O* Instant) 110
oats (*Quaker* Quick/Old Fashioned), 1/2 cup 150
oats, all varieties, except almond raisin (*H-O* Explo
Instant) 170
oats, almond raisin (*H-O* Explo Instant) 160
oats, apple and cinnamon (*H-O* Instant) 130
oats, maple and brown sugar (*H-O* Instant) 160
oats, toasted (*H-O* Old Fashioned), 1/3 cup 160
rye, cream of (*Roman Meal* Instant) 100
wheat (*Wheatena*), 1/3 cup 150

Cereal, cooking *(cont.)*
wheat, all varieties (*Malt-O-Meal/Malt-O-Meal* Quick), 3 tbsp. 120
wheat, farina (*H-O*), 3 tbsp. 120
Cereal bar, see "Granola and cereal bar"
Chayote:
fresh, raw (*Frieda's*), 3.5 oz. 28
boiled, drained, 1″ pieces, ½ cup 19
Cheese (see also "Cheese food" and "Cheese product"):
American, processed (*Old English* Loaf), 1 oz. 100
American, processed (*Old English* Slice), 1-oz. slice . . . 110
(*Bel Paese*) medalions, ¾ oz. 65
blue, crumbled (*Sargento*), ¼ cup, 1 oz. 100
Brie, 1 oz. 95
butterkase, plain or smoked (*Boar's Head*), 1 oz. 100
Camembert, 1 oz. 85
cheddar (*Boar's Head* Double Glouster), 1 oz. 110
cheddar, lower fat (*Alpine Lace* Reduced Fat), 1 oz. 80
cheddar, mild, sharp, or extra sharp (*Heluva* Good), 1 oz. 110
cheddar, sharp (*Boar's Head* Slicing), 1 oz. 110
cheddar, sharp (*Sargento* Sliced), 1 oz. 110
cheddar, shredded, mild (*Sargento Preferred Light*), ¼ cup 70
cheddar, shredded, mild or sharp (*Sargento*), ¼ cup . . . 110
Cheshire, 1 oz. 110
Colby (*Sargento* Sliced), 1 oz. 110
Colby, lower fat (*Alpine Lace* Reduced Fat), 1 oz. 80
Colby, mild (*Heluva* Good Longhorn), 1 oz. 117
Colby-Jack (*Heluva* Good), 1 oz. 110
Colby-Jack, shredded (*Sargento*), ¼ cup 110
cottage, 4% fat (*Breakstone's/Sealtest*), ½ cup 120
cottage, dry curd (*Breakstone's*), ¼ cup 45
cottage, 2% fat (*Breakstone's/Sealtest*) ½ cup 9
cottage, 1% fat (*Light n' Lively*) ½ cup 80
cream cheese (*Philadelphia Brand*), 1 oz. 100
cream cheese, with chives or pimiento (*Philadelphia Brand*), 1 oz. 90
cream cheese, fat free (*Philadelphia Brand*), 1 oz. 25

cream cheese, soft (*Philadelphia Brand*), 2 tbsp.:
- plain 100
- plain, fat free 30
- plain, light 70
- with chives and onion or herb and garlic 110
- with olive and pimiento or smoked salmon 100
- with pineapple or strawberries 100

cream cheese, whipped (*Philadelphia Brand*), 3 tbsp.:
- plain 110
- with smoked salmon 100

Edam (*Boar's Head*), 1 oz. 90
farmer (*Western Creamy*), 2.3 oz. 100
farmer, dry (*Western Creamy* Fat Free), 2 oz. 50
feta, (*Classika* Portions), 1 oz. 100
feta, lower fat (*Alpine Lace* Reduced Fat), 1 oz. 60
fontina (*Classica*), 1 oz. 110
goat, hard type, 1 oz. 128
goat, semisoft type, 1 oz. 103
goat, soft type, 1 oz. 76
Gorgonzola (*Galbani* Dolcelatte), 1 oz. 93
Gouda (*Boar's Head*), 1 oz. 110
Gruyère, 1 oz. 117
Havarti (*Boar's Head*), 1 oz. 110
Italian (*Classica Italiana*), 1 oz. 110
Italian style, shredded (*Sargento Recipe Blend*), 1/4 cup . . . 90
Jarlsberg (*Sargento*), 1.2-oz. slice 120
(*Laughing Cow Babybel* 7 oz.), 1 oz. 100
(*Laughing Cow Babybel* Mini), 3/4-oz. piece 70
(*Laughing Cow* Original Wedge), 1 oz. 70
Limburger (*Kraft Mohawk Valley*), 1 oz. 90
mascarpone (*Classica* Domestic), 1 oz. 120
mascarpone (*Galbani* Imported), 1 oz. 140
Mexican, 4, shredded (*Sargento Recipe Blend*), 1/4 cup . . 110
Monterey Jack (*Sargento* Sliced), 1 oz. 100
Monterey Jack, regular or with jalapeño (*Boar's Head*), 1 oz. 100
Monterey Jack, regular or with jalapeño (*Heluva* Good), 1 oz. 100
Monterey Jack, shredded (*Sargento*), 1/4 cup 100

Cheese ***(cont.)***

mozzarella (*Boar's Head*), 1 oz. 90
mozzarella, whole milk (*Heluva* Good), 1 oz. 80
mozzarella, part skim (*Alpine Lace* Reduced Fat), 1 oz. . . . 70
mozzarella, part skim (*Heluva* Good), 1 oz. 70
mozzarella, sliced (*Sargento*), 1.6-oz. slice 130
mozzarella, sliced, light (*Sargento Preferred Light*), 1.6 oz. 90
mozzarella, shredded (*Sargento*), 1/4 cup 80
mozzarella, shredded, light (*Sargento Preferred Light*), 1/4 cup 70
Muenster (*Boar's Head*), 1 oz. 100
Muenster (*Heluva* Good), 1 oz. 100
Muenster, sliced (*Sargento* Sliced), 1 oz. 100
Neufchâtel (*Philadelphia Brand*), 1 oz. 70
Parmesan, grated (*Sargento*), 1 tbsp. 25
Parmesan, grated or shredded (*Classica*), 1 tbsp. 20
Parmesan, shredded (*Sargento*), 1/4 cup 110
Parmesan and Romano, grated (*Sargento*), 1 tbsp. 25
Parmesan and Romano, shredded (*Sargento*), 1/4 cup . . . 110
pimiento, processed (*Kraft* Deluxe), 1 oz. 100
pizza, shredded (*Sargento/Sargento Pizza Double Cheese*), 1/4 cup 90
Port du Salut, 1 oz. 100
provolone (*Boar's Head*), 1 oz. 100
provolone, lower fat (*Alpine Lace* Reduced Fat), 1 oz. . . . 70
provolone, sliced (*Sargento* Sliced), 1 oz. 100
ricotta (*Sargento* Old Fashioned), 1/4 cup 90
ricotta, part skim (*Sargento*), 1 oz. 80
ricotta, light (*Sargento* Light), 1/4 cup 60
Romano, grated, dry or fresh (*Classica* Pecorino), 1 tbsp. 20
Romano, shredded (*Classica* Pecorino), 1 tbsp. 20
Roquefort, 1 oz. 105
string, snack (*MooTown Snackers*), 1 piece, .8 oz. 70
string, snack, light (*MooTown Snackers*), .8 oz. 60
Swiss (*Boar's Head* Domestic), 1 oz. 100
Swiss (*Boar's Head* Gold Label Imported/No Salt), 1 oz. 110
Swiss, lower fat (*Alpine Lace* Reduced Fat), 1 oz. 90

Swiss, sliced (*Sargento* Sliced), 3/4-oz. slice 80
Swiss, sliced, light (*Sargento Preferred Light* Sliced),
1 oz. 80
Swiss, shredded (*Sargento*), 1/4 cup 110
taco or nacho and taco, shredded (*Sargento*), 1/4 cup . . . 110
taco, light (*Sargento Preferred Light*), 1/4 cup 70
"Cheese," substitute and nondairy:
all varieties (*Smart Beat*), 2/3-oz. slice 25
cheddar flavor, shredded (*Sargento*), 1/4 cup 90
cream, all varieties (*Tofutti Better Than Cream Cheese*),
1 oz. 80
mozzarella, shredded (*Sargento*), 1/4 cup 80
Cheese dip, 2 tbsp.:
(*Chi-Chi's* Fiesta) 40
bacon (*Nalley's*) 110
cheddar, mild (*Old Dutch*) 30
cheddar, jalapeño and (*Breakstone's*) 60
cheddar and mustard (*Heluva* Good Pretzel) 80
nacho (*Old Dutch*) 35
nacho (*Nalley's*) 120
nacho, mild (*Guiltless Gourmet*) 25
Parmesan garlic (*Marie's*) 140
salsa (*Heluva* Good Cheese 'N Salsa) 80
Cheese dip, mix, nacho (*Knorr*), 1/2 tsp. 10
Cheese food (see also "Cheese"):
all varieties (*Kaukauna*), 1 oz. 90
all varieties (*Kaukauna* Premium Blend), 1 oz. 100
all varieties, light (*Kaukauna Lite 50*), 1 oz. 70
all varieties (*Kraft* Singles), 3/4-oz. slice 70
all varieties, shredded (*Velveeta/Velveeta* Mexican),
1/4 cup 130
American (*Heluva* Good), 1 oz. 70
American, grated (*Kraft*), 1 tbsp. 25
Cheese nut log, sharp (*Wispride*), 2 tbsp. 100
Cheese product:
(*Cheez Whiz Light*), 2 tbsp. 80
(*Velveeta Light*), 1 oz. 60
all varieties (*Kraft Free* Singles), 3/4-oz. slice 30
all varieties (*Alpine Lace* Fat Free), 1 oz. 45

American flavor (*Alpine Lace*), 1 oz. 80
Cheese sandwich, frozen, grilled (*Swanson Fun Feast*), 1 pkg. 460
Cheese sauce, 2 tbsp.:
(*Cheez Whiz* Squeezable) 100
(*Cheez Whiz Zap-A-Pack)* 90
all varieties (*Kaukauna Micro Melt*) 80
nacho (*Kaukauna*) 80
salsa (*Cheez Whiz Zap-A-Pack)* 90
Cheese sauce mix:
(*French's*), 1/4 pkg. 25
four (*Knorr*), 1/3 pkg. 70
nacho (*Durkee*), 1/5 pkg. 25
Cheese spread, 2 tbsp., except as noted:
all flavors (*Cheez Whiz*) 90
all flavors (*Velveeta/Velveeta Italiana/Velveeta*Mexican), 1 oz. 80
American, with bacon (*Kraft*) 90
blue cheese (*Kraft Roka*) 80
cheddar, sharp, or with bacon or horseradish (*Heluva* Good) 90
Limburger (*Mohawk Valley*) 80
Neufchâtel, all varieties (*Kaukauna*), 1 oz. 80
olive and pimiento (*Kraft*) 70
pimiento (*Kraft*) 80
pineapple (*Kraft*) 70
port wine (*Heluva* Good) 90
sharp (*Old English*) 90
slices (*Velveeta*), 3/4 oz. 60
Cheese stick, cornmeal coated (*Goya*Surullitos), 7 pieces 300
Cheeseburger, see "Beef sandwich"
Cheesecake, see "Cake, frozen"
Cherimoya (see also "Custard apple"):
fresh, 1 medium, 1.9 lb. 515
fresh (*Frieda's*), 3.5 oz. 94
Cherries jubilee (*Lucky Leaf/Musselman's*), 1/4 cup 80
Cherry, 1/2 cup, except as noted:
fresh, sour, red, with pits 26

fresh, sour, red, pitted 39
fresh, sweet, with pits 52
canned, sour, red, pitted, in water (*Lucky Leaf/ Musselman's*) 60
canned, sweet, pitted, in syrup (*S&W/S&W* Royal Anne) 140
dried, bing, pitted (*Frieda's*), 1 oz. 79
frozen, sour, red, unsweetened, pitted, 4 oz. 52
frozen, sweet, sweetened, pitted, 4 oz. 101

Cherry, candied, green or red:
(*S&W* Glace), 5 pieces 80
and pineapple mix (*Paradise/White Swan*), 2 tbsp., 1.3 oz. 110

Cherry, maraschino, green or red (*S&W*), 1 piece 10

Cherry drink:
blend (*Tree Top* Not Plain Cherry), 8 fl. oz. 120
wild (*Capri Sun*), 6.75 fl. oz. 110

Cherry juice, 8 fl. oz.:
(*After the Fall* Very Cherry) 100
(*Juicy Juice*) 130
black (*Heinke's/R.W. Knudsen*) 180

Cherry juice blend, 8 fl. oz.:
(*Dole* Mountain) 120
(*Veryfine* Juice-Ups) 150
black (*R.W. Knudsen* Concentrate) 130
cider (*R.W. Knudsen*) 130

Cherry nectar (*Santa Cruz*), 8 fl. oz. 110

Cherry pastry, dumpling, frozen (*Pepperidge Farm*) 1 piece 280

Chestnut, European, roasted, peeled, 1 oz. 70

Chicken, fresh, 4 oz., except as noted:
broiler-fryer, roasted:
with skin, ½ chicken, 10.5 oz. (15.8 oz. with bone) . . 715
with skin 271
meat only 215
meat only, chopped or diced, 1 cup 266
dark meat only 232
light meat only 196
breast, with skin, ½ breast, 3.5 oz. (8.5 oz. with bone) 193

Chicken, broiler-fryer, roasted *(cont.)*
drumstick, with skin, 1.8 oz. (2.9 oz. with bone) . . . 112
leg, with skin (5.7 oz. with bone) 265
thigh, with skin, 2.2 oz. (2.9 oz. with bone) 153
wing, with skin, 1.2 oz. (2.3 oz. with bone) 99
capon, roasted, with skin, ½ capon, 1.4 lbs. (2 lbs. with bone) 1457
capon, with skin 260
roaster, roasted, with skin, ½ chicken, 1 lb. (1.5 lbs. with bone) 1071
roaster, roasted, with skin 253
stewing, stewed:
with skin, ½ chicken, 9.2 oz. (13.5 oz. with bone) . . 744
with skin 323
meat only 269
meat only, chopped or diced, 1 cup 332
Chicken, canned, chunk, 2 oz. or ¼ cup:
breast (*Hormel/Hormel* No Salt) 60
regular or regular in water (*Swanson/Swanson* Premium) . 90
in broth (*Swanson* Mixin') 110
white or white in water (*Swanson/Swanson* Premium) . . . 80
Chicken, ground:
raw (*Perdue/Perdue* Burger), 4 oz. 180
cooked (*Perdue/Perdue* Burger), 3 oz. 170
Chicken, refrigerated or frozen:
whole, cooked, dark meat (*Perdue*), 3 oz. 210
whole, cooked, dark meat (*Perdue Oven Stuffer*), 3 oz. . . 200
whole, cooked, white meat (*Perdue/Perdue Oven Stuffer*), 3 oz. 160
breast, raw, halves (*Tyson*), 4 oz. 190
breast, raw, halves, skinless (*Tyson*), 4 oz. 130
breast, raw, quarters (*Tyson*), 4 oz. 210
breast, raw, boneless (*Perdue/Perdue Oven Stuffer*), 4 oz. 130
breast, raw, boneless tenderloins (*Tyson*), 4 oz. 110
breast, cooked, whole (*Perdue*), 3 oz. 160
breast, cooked, whole (*Perdue Oven Stuffer*), 3 oz. 150

breast, cooked, boneless (*Perdue/Perdue Oven Stuffer*), 3 oz. 120
breast, cooked, quartered (*Perdue*), 3 oz. 180
breast, cooked, roundelet (*Tyson*), 2.6-oz. piece 170
breast, cooked, tenderloins (*Perdue*), 3 oz. 100
breast, roasted (*Tyson*), ½ breast 250
breast, roasted (*Chicken By George*), 4 oz. 110
breast, roasted, boneless (*Perdue*), 3.6-oz. half 140
breast, roasted, skinless (*Perdue*), 5.9-oz. half 250
breast, roasted, seasoned, 4 oz.:
  Cajun or garlic and herb (*Chicken By George*) 120
  Caribbean grill (*Chicken By George*) 150
  Italian bleu cheese, lemon oregano, or teriyaki (*Chicken By George*) 130
  lemon herb or mesquite barbecue (*Chicken By George*) 120
  mustard dill or tomato herb basil (*Chicken By George*) 140
diced (*Tyson*), 9 oz. 130
drumstick, roasted (*Perdue*), 2.2-oz. piece 110
drumstick, roasted (*Perdue Oven Stuffer*), 3.6-oz. piece 190
drumstick, roasted (*Tyson*), 3 pieces 330
drumstick, roasted, skinless (*Perdue* Pick), 2 pieces, 3.5 oz. 150
leg, whole, roasted (*Perdue*), 5.5-oz. leg 370
leg, quarters, raw (*Tyson*), 4 oz. 230
leg, quarters, cooked (*Perdue*), 3 oz. 210
thigh, raw (*Tyson*), 4 oz. 250
thigh, raw, boneless, skinless (*Tyson*), 4 oz. 160
thigh, roasted (*Perdue*), 3.2-oz. piece 240
thigh, roasted, boneless (*Perdue*), 2 thighs, 3.6 oz. 200
thigh, roasted, boneless (*Perdue Oven Stuffer*), 3.3-oz. piece 170
thigh, roasted, skinless (*Tyson*), 3-oz. thigh 160
wing, raw, whole (*Tyson*), 4 oz. 250
wing, roasted (*Perdue*), 2 wings, 3.2 oz. 210
Chicken dinner, frozen, 1 pkg.:
barbecue, mesquite (*Healthy Choice*) 320
boneless (*Swanson Hungry Man*) 690

Chicken dinner *(cont.)*
breaded, country (*Healthy Choice*) 350
broccoli Alfredo (*Healthy Choice*) 370
Cantonese (*Healthy Choice*) 210
Dijon (*Healthy Choice*) 280
fried (*Banquet* Extra Helping) 790
fried, country, gravy (*Marie Callender's*) 610
fried, dark (*Swanson*) 550
fried, dark (*Swanson* Budget) 460
fried, dark (*Swanson Hungry Man*) 810
fried, Southern (*Banquet* Extra Helping) 750
fried, white (*Banquet* Extra Helping) 820
fried, white (*Swanson*) 560
fried, white, mostly (*Swanson Hungry Man*) 810
glazed, Southwestern (*Healthy Choice*) 300
grilled, patties (*Swanson Hungry Man*) 580
grilled, white, in garlic sauce (*Swanson*) 260
herb, country (*Healthy Choice*) 270
nuggets (*Swanson*) 440
parmigiana (*Banquet* Extra Helping) 650
parmigiana (*Healthy Choice*) 300
parmigiana (*Marie Callender's*) 620
parmigiana (*Swanson*) 400
parmigiana (*Swanson* Budget) 340
pasta and (*Swanson* Budget) 250
picante (*Healthy Choice*) 220
with rice (*Goya* Arroz Con Pollo) 750
roasted, herb (*Swanson*) 290
roasted, herb, mashed potatoes (*Marie Callender's*) 670
sweet and sour (*Healthy Choice*) 310
tenders, platter (*Swanson*) 320
teriyaki (*Healthy Choice*) 270

Chicken entree, canned:
à la king (*Swanson* Main Dish), 1 cup 320
à la king (*Top Shelf*), 10 oz. 380
breast, glazed (*Top Shelf*), 10 oz. 200
and broccoli (*Healthy Choice Hearty Handfuls*), 6.1 oz. . . 320
cacciatore (*Top Shelf*), 10 oz. 210
chow mein (*La Choy* Bi-Pack), 1 cup 110

chow mein (*La Choy* Entree), 1 cup 80
and dumplings (*Swanson* Main Dish), 1 cup 260
Oriental, with noodles (*La Choy*), 1 cup 150
spicy (*La Choy* Szechuan Bi-Pack), 1 cup 100
stew (*Swanson* Main Dish), 1 cup 180
sweet and sour (*La Choy* Bi-Pack), 1 cup 160
teriyaki (*La Choy* Bi-Pack), 1 cup 110

Chicken entree, frozen, (see also "Chicken entree, refrigerated"):

à la king (*Banquet* Toppers), 4.5-oz. bag 100
à la king (*Stouffer's*), 9½ oz. 320
Alfredo (*Stouffer's Lunch Express*), 9⅝ oz. 360
baked, and gravy, whipped potato (*Stouffer's* Homestyle), 8⅞ oz. 270
baked, whipped potato (*Lean Cuisine*), 8⅝ oz. 250
barbecue, glazed (*Weight Watchers*), 9 oz. 230
barbecue, honey, with potato, vegetables (*Tyson*), 11 oz. 430
barbecue, with potato, vegetables (*Tyson* BBQ), 11 oz. . . 360
barbecue style (*Banquet*), 9 oz. 320
biryani (*Curry Classics*), 10 oz. 460
blackened (*Tyson*), 9 oz. 260
breaded cutlet, pasta marinara and (*Celentano*), 10 oz. . . 170
breast, breaded (*Tyson*), 2 fillets, 3 oz. 180
breast, breaded, Southern (*Tyson Breast Fillets*), 2 fillets, 3 oz. 170
breast, in wine sauce (*Lean Cuisine* Cafe Classics), 8⅛ oz. 220
breast tenders (*Banquet*), 3 pieces, 3 oz. 260
breast tenders (*Tyson*), 5 pieces, 3 oz. 210
breast tenders, Southern (*Banquet*), 3 pieces, 3 oz. 260
with broccoli and cheese (*Tyson*), 9 oz. 260
cacciatore (*Healthy Choice*), 12.5 oz. 260
calypso (*Lean Cuisine* Cafe Classics), 8.5 oz. 280
carbonara (*Lean Cuisine* Cafe Classics), 9 oz. 290
chow mein (*Banquet*), 9 oz. 210
chow mein (*Chun King*), 13 oz. 370
chow mein (*Lean Cuisine*), 9 oz. 210
chow mein (*Stouffer's Lunch Express*), 10⅝ oz. 260

Chicken entree, frozen *(cont.)*
chunks, breaded:
(*Country Skillet*), 5 pieces, 3.3 oz. 270
(*Tyson Breast Chunks*), 6 pieces, 3 oz. 220
(*Tyson Chick'n Chunks*), 6 pieces, 3 oz. 280
and cheddar (*Banquet*), 4 pieces, 2.9 oz. 280
Southern (*Banquet*), 5 pieces, 3.1 oz. 270
Southern (*Country Skillet*), 5 pieces, 3.3 oz. 250
Southern (*Tyson Chick'n Chunks*), 6 pieces, 3 oz. . . . 250
Cordon Bleu (*Weight Watchers*), 9 oz. 230
creamed (*Stouffer's*), 6½ oz. 280
creamy, and broccoli (*Stouffer's*), 8⅞ oz. 320
croquettes (*Goya*), 3 pieces 280
and dumplings (*Banquet* Homestyle), 10 oz. 260
enchilada, see "Enchilada entree"
escalloped, and noodles (*Stouffer's*), 10 oz. 450
fettuccini (*Lean Cuisine*), 9 oz. 270
fettuccini (*Stouffer's* Homestyle), 10½ oz. 390
fettuccini (*Weight Watchers*), 10 oz. 290
fettuccini Alfredo (*Healthy Choice*), 8.5 oz. 260
fettuccini, with broccoli (*Lean Cuisine Lunch Express*),
10¼ oz. 290
fiesta (*Lean Cuisine*), 8.5 oz. 260
Français (*Tyson*), 9 oz. 260
Francesca (*Healthy Choice*), 12.5 oz. 360
fried:
(*Banquet* Original Meal), 9 oz. 470
(*Morton*), 9 oz. 420
Southern (*Banquet* Meal), 8.75 oz. 530
whipped potatoes (*Stouffer's* Homestyle), 7⅛ oz. . . . 330
whipped potatoes (*Swanson*), 1 pkg. 400
white meat (*Banquet* Meal), 8.75 oz. 470
fried, pieces:
(*Banquet* Original), 3 oz. 270
(*Country Skillet*), 3 oz. 270
breast (*Banquet Original*), 5.5-oz. piece 410
country (*Banquet*), 3 oz. 270
drums and thighs (*Banquet*), 3 oz. 260
honey BBQ, skinless (*Banquet*), 3 oz. 210

hot 'n spicy (*Banquet*), 3 oz. 260
skinless (*Banquet*), 3 oz. 210
Southern (*Banquet*), 3 oz. 270
wings, hot and spicy (*Banquet*), 4 oz., 4 pieces 230
fried rice (*Tyson* Kit), 1 cup 200
garlic (*Healthy Choice Hearty Handfuls*), 6.1 oz. 330
garlic, Milano (*Healthy Choice*), 9.5 oz. 240
ginger, Hunan (*Healthy Choice*), 12.6 oz. 350
glazed, country (*Healthy Choice*), 8.5 oz. 200
glazed, with rice, broccoli, and carrots (*Tyson*), 9.25 oz. 240
glazed, with vegetable rice (*Lean Cuisine*), 8.5 oz. 240
grilled, and angel-hair pasta (*Stouffer's Lunch Express*), 9 7/8 oz. 340
grilled, with corn, beans (*Tyson*), 7.75 oz. 220
grilled, Italian, with linguini (*Tyson*), 9 oz. 190
grilled, salsa (*Lean Cuisine* Cafe Classics), 8 7/8 oz. 240
gumbo (*Goya* Asopao de Pollo), 11 oz. 190
herb, with radiatore, vegetables (*Tyson*), 11.5 oz. 320
honey mustard (*Healthy Choice*), 9.5 oz. 260
honey mustard (*Lean Cuisine* Cafe Classics), 8 oz. 270
honey mustard (*Smart Ones*), 8.5 oz. 200
honey mustard, with gemelli (*Tyson*), 11.5 oz. 330
imperial (*Healthy Choice*), 9 oz. 230
Italian, with fettuccini (*Lean Cuisine*), 9 oz. 270
Kiev (*Tyson*), 9.25 oz. 440
with linguine (*Stouffer's Lunch Express*), 9 5/8 oz. 300
lo mein (*Banquet*), 10.5 oz. 270
mandarin (*Healthy Choice*), 10 oz. 280
mandarin (*Lean Cuisine Lunch Express*), 9 3/4 oz. 270
marinara, with pasta (*Tyson*), 11.5 oz. 430
Marsala, with potato, carrots (*Tyson*), 9 oz. 180
Marsala, and vegetables (*Healthy Choice*), 11.5 oz. 220
Mediterranean (*Lean Cuisine* Cafe Classics), 10 1/8 oz. . . . 250
mesquite (*Tyson*), 9 oz. 310
Mexican, and rice (*Stouffer's Lunch Express*), 9 1/8 oz. . . 280
Mirabella (*Smart Ones*), 9.2 oz. 170
Monterey (*Stouffer's* Homestyle), 9 3/8 oz. 410
and mushroom (*Healthy Choice Hearty Handfuls*), 6.1 oz. 300
with mushroom sauce (*Tyson*), 9 oz. 220

Chicken entree, frozen *(cont.)*

nibbles (*Swanson*), 1 pkg. 340
and noodles (*Stouffer's* Homestyle), 10 oz. 300
noodle casserole (*Swanson*), 1 pkg. 290
noodle casserole, with vegetables (*Swanson*), 1 pkg. . . . 320
nuggets (*Banquet*), 6 pieces, 3 oz. 240
nuggets (*Banquet*), 6 pieces, 4.5 oz. 320
nuggets (*Banquet* Homestyle), 6.75 oz. 410
nuggets (*Country Skillet*), 10 pieces, 3.3 oz. 280
nuggets (*Morton*), 7 oz. 320
nuggets, mozzarella (*Banquet*), 6 pieces, 2.9 oz. 250
nuggets, Southern (*Banquet*), 6 pieces, 4.5 oz. 340
à la orange (*Lean Cuisine*), 9 oz. 260
Oriental (*Banquet*), 9 oz. 260
Oriental (*Lean Cuisine*), 9 oz. 260
Oriental (*Stouffer's Lunch Express*), 9¾ oz. 370
Parmesan (*Lean Cuisine* Cafe Classics), 10⅞ oz. 240
parmigiana (*Banquet*), 9.5 oz. 290
parmigiana (*Banquet* Family Size), 4.7-oz. patty 240
parmigiana (*Stouffer's* Homestyle), 10⅞ oz. 320
parmigiana (*Tyson*), 10.8 oz. 290
parmigiana (*Weight Watchers*), 10 oz. 310
parmigiana, Italian style (*Banquet*), 4.6-oz. patty 250
patties, breaded:
  (*Banquet*), 2.3-oz. patty 180
  (*Banquet*), 10.2 oz. 380
  (*Country Skillet*), 2.5-oz. patty 190
  (*Morton*), 6.75 oz. 280
  (*Tyson Thick'n Crispy*), 2.5-oz. patty 200
  breast (*Tyson*), 2.5-oz. patty 190
  breast, Southern (*Tyson*), 2.5-oz. patty 180
  with cheddar (*Tyson Chick'n with Cheddar*), 2.5-oz. patty 220
  Southern (*Banquet*), 2.3-oz. patty 170
  Southern (*Country Skillet*), 3.3-oz. patty 190
  Southern (*Tyson Chick'n Chunks*), 6 pieces, 3 oz. . . . 250
in peanut sauce (*Lean Cuisine*), 9 oz. 280
penne pollo (*Weight Watchers*), 10 oz. 290
piccata (*Lean Cuisine* Cafe Classics), 9 oz. 290

piccata, with potato, broccoli (*Tyson*), 9 oz. 180
pie or pot pie:
(*Banquet*), 7 oz. 350
(*Empire* Kosher), 8.2 oz. 440
(*Lean Cuisine*), 9.5 oz. 320
(*Marie Callender's*), 10-oz. pie 680
(*Stouffer's*), 10 oz. 560
(*Swanson*), 1 pkg. 410
(*Swanson* Deluxe), 1 pkg. 470
(*Swanson Hungry Man*), 1 pkg. 650
(*Tyson* Meat Lovers), 9 oz. 600
au gratin (*Marie Callender's*), 10-oz. pie 720
and broccoli (*Marie Callender's*), 10-oz. pie 780
broccoli and cheese (*Tyson*), 9 oz. 580
and vegetables (*Tyson*), 9 oz. 550
primavera, with pasta (*Banquet*), 10.5 oz. 330
primavera, with pasta (*Tyson*), 11.5 oz. 390
and rice, stir-fry casserole (*Swanson*), 1 pkg. 240
roast, glazed (*Weight Watchers*), 9.3 oz. 240
roasted, herb (*Lean Cuisine* Cafe Classics), 8 oz. 210
roasted, with linguini, broccoli (*Tyson*), 9 oz. 190
sandwich, see "Chicken sandwich"
sesame (*Healthy Choice*), 9.75 oz. 240
sesame, Shanghai (*Healthy Choice*), 12 oz. 310
stir-fry (*Tyson* Kit), 1 cup 180
strips, breaded (*Swanson*), 1 pkg. 340
supreme, with potato, green beans (*Tyson*), 9 oz. 230
tikka (*Curry Classics* Makhanwala), 10 oz. 480
and vegetables (*Lean Cuisine*), 10½ oz. 240
with vegetables, garden (*Stouffer's Lunch Express*),
9⅞ oz. 340
walnut, crunchy (*Chun King*), 13 oz. 470
wings, barbecue (*Tyson*), 4 pieces 220
wings, teriyaki (*Tyson*), 4 pieces 190
Chicken entree, mix*, stir-fried (*Tyson*), 1 cup 150
Chicken entree, refrigerated (see also "Chicken, refrigerated or frozen"):
all varieties except nuggets (*Perdue Short Cuts*), 3 oz. . . 110
cutlet, breaded (*Perdue* Original), 3.5-oz. piece 230

Chicken entree, refrigerated *(cont.)*
nuggets, breaded (*Perdue* Original), 5 pieces, 3 oz. 200
nuggets, breaded, and cheese (*Perdue*), 5 pieces, 3 oz. 220
oven roasted, dark meat (*Perdue*), 3 oz. 170
oven roasted, white meat (*Perdue*), 3 oz. 140
tenderloins, breaded (*Perdue* Original), 3 oz. 160
wings, barbecued (*Perdue*), 3 oz. 200
wings, hot and spicy (*Perdue*), 3 oz. 190
Chicken fat, rendered (*Empire* Kosher), 1 tbsp. 120
Chicken frankfurter (*Empire* Kosher), 2-oz. link 100
Chicken giblets, simmered, chopped, 1 cup 228
Chicken gravy, 1/4 cup:
(*Franco-American*) 45
(*Heinz* Home Style Classic) 20
cream of (*Pepperidge Farm*) 30
giblet (*Franco-American*) 30
golden, with chicken, or rotisserie flavor (*Pepperidge Farm*) 25
mix* (*Durkee*) 20
mix*, roasted (*Knorr*) 30
Chicken lunch meat:
breast, oven roasted (*Boar's Head* Golden), 2 oz. 50
breast (*Hebrew National*), 2 oz. 45
breast, peppered or smoked (*Tyson*), 3 slices, 2.2 oz. . . . 50
breast, smoked (*Boar's Head* Hickory), 2 oz. 60
white, sliced (*Tyson*), 3 slices 90
Chicken sandwich, frozen, 1 piece:
(*Hormel Quick Meal*) 340
grilled (*Hormel Quick Meal*) 300
pastry (*Mrs. Paterson's Aussie Pie*) 460
pocket, and cheddar with broccoli (*Hot Pockets*) 300
pocket, fajita or Parmesan (*Lean Pockets*) 260
pocket, glazed, supreme (*Lean Pockets*) 240
Chicken sauce:
barbecue flavor (*Hunt's Chicken Sensations*), 1 tbsp. 35
Caesar, crispy (*Lawry's*), 2 tbsp. 30
Italian garlic or lemon herb (*Hunt's Chicken Sensations*), 1 tbsp. 30
sherried (*Lawry's*), 1 tbsp. 20

Southwestern (*Hunt's Chicken Sensations*), 1 tbsp. 30
Thai, satay (*Lawry's*), 1 tbsp. 35
wing, hot or mild (*Nance's*) 2 tbsp. 15
Chicken sausage, 3.3-oz. link:
and apricot or sundried tomato with basil (*Bilinski*) 120
and broccoli or pesto (*Bilinski*) 110
Italian, with pepper and onion (*Bilinski*) 120
and jalapeño (*Bilinski*) 130
and spinach (*Bilinski*) 100
Chicken seasoning and coating mix, 1/8 pkg., except as noted:
(*Shake 'n Bake* Original Recipe) 40
barbecue glaze (*Shake 'n Bake*) 45
Buffalo wing, Cajun or garlic and herb (*Durkee*) 15
Buffalo wing, hot, mild, or screaming hot (*Durkee*) 20
coq au vin (*Knorr* Recipe), 1 tbsp. 30
extra crispy (*Oven Fry*) 60
homestyle flour (*Oven Fry*) 40
hot and spicy (*Shake 'n Bake*) 40
Southwest, marinade (*Lawry's*), 1 tsp. 5
Chicken spread:
chunky (*Underwood*), 1/4 cup 120
salad (*Libby's Spreadables*), 1/3 cup 140
Chick-fil-A, 1 serving:
chicken:
plain, no bun, .7 oz. 160
chargrilled, 2.8 oz. 130
Chick-fil-A Nuggets, 8-pack 290
Chick-n-Strips, 4 pcs. 230
Chick-n-Strips salad 290
salad, chargrilled garden 170
salad plate 290
chicken sandwiches:
regular 290
chargrilled 280
chargrilled, deluxe 290
chargrilled club, without dressing 390
Chick-n-Q 370
deluxe 300

Chick-fil-A,* chicken sandwiches *(cont.)
salad, whole wheat 320
side dishes, small:
carrot-raisin salad 150
chicken soup, 1 cup 110
coleslaw 130
tossed salad 70
Waffle fries, salted or unsalted 290
desserts:
brownie, fudge nut 350
cheesecake 270
cheesecake, blueberry or strawberry 290
Icedream, small cone 140
Icedream, small cup 350
lemon pie 280
Chickpeas:
dry (*Arrowhead Mills*), 1/4 cup 170
dry, boiled, 1/2 cup 134
canned (*Allens/East Texas Fair*), 1/2 cup 120
canned (*Stokely*), 1/2 cup 110
canned, in tomato sauce (*Goya*), 1/2 cup 100
Chicory, witloof, 1/2 cup 8
Chicory greens, chopped, 1/2 cup 21
Chicory root, 1" pieces, 1/2 cup 33
Chili, canned, 1 cup, except as noted:
with beans (*Gebhardt*) 320
with beans (*Libby's*) 420
with beans (*Libby's Diner*), 7 3/4 oz. 320
with beans (*Nalley* Real Hearty) 310
with beans (*Nalley* Thick) 290
with beans, regular or hot (*Hormel*) 340
with beans, chunky (*Hormel*) 330
without beans (*Libby's*) 480
without beans (*Nalley* Big Chunk) 280
without beans, regular or jalapeño (*Wolf*) 420
without beans, onion (*Nalley* Walla Walla) 300
without beans, regular or hot (*Hormel*) 410
with macaroni (*Hormel* Chili Mac), 7 1/2-oz. can 200
turkey, with beans (*Hormel*) 220

turkey, without beans (*Hormel*) 190
vegetarian (*Hormel*) 200
Chili, frozen:
with beans (*Stouffer's* Entree), 8¾ oz. 270
with corn bread (*Marie Callender's* Dinner), 16 oz. 350
three bean (*Lean Cuisine* Entree), 9 oz. 210
Chili, mix*:
4 bean (*Knorr* Cup), 1 pkg. 230
3 bean or vegetarian (*Spice Islands* Quick Meal), 1 pkg. 180
Chili base, canned:
(*Hunt's* Homestyle Fixings) ½ cup 85
all varieties (*S&W* Chili Makin's), ½ cup 80
Chili beans (see also "Mexican beans"), canned, ½ cup:
(*Hunt's*) 85
(*S&W*) 110
hot (*S&W* Chipotle) 90
zesty sauce (*Campbell's*) 130
Chili dip, green (*La Victoria*), 2 tbsp. 10
Chili dip mix, caliente (*Knorr*), ½ tsp. 5
Chili pepper, see "Pepper, chili"
Chili powder, 1 tbsp. 24
Chili sauce (see also "Pepper sauce" and "Szechuan sauce"):
(*Nance's*), 2 tbsp. 25
(*S&W* Steakhouse), 1 tbsp. 15
hot dog (*Just Rite*), 2 oz. 50
Chili seasoning mix:
(*Durkee* Pot-O), ⅛ pkg. 30
(*Lawry's*), 1 tbsp. 25
(*Lawry's* Tex-Mex), 2 tbsp. 50
(*Mick Fowler's 2-Alarm* Kit), 3 tbsp. 60
(*Mick Fowler's 2-Alarm* Family), 2 tbsp. 50
mild (*Durkee*), ⅕ pkg. 30
Texas red (*Durkee*), ⅓ pkg. 45
Chimichanga, frozen:
beefsteak and bean (*Don Miguel*), 7 oz. 410
chicken (*Don Miguel*), 7 oz. 400
Chimichanga dinner, frozen:
beef (*Chi-Chi's*), 15 oz. 630

chicken (*Chi-Chi's* Chix), 15 oz. 600
Chimichanga entree, frozen (*Banquet*), 9.5 oz. 470
Chitterlings, pork, simmered, 4 oz. 344
Chives, fresh, chopped, or freeze-dried, 1 tbsp. 1
Chocolate, see "Candy"
Chocolate, baking:
bar, milk (*Ghirardelli*), 1 oz. 142
bar, semisweet (*Baker's*), 1 oz. 130
bar, sweet (*Baker's German*), ½ oz. 60
bar, unsweetened (*Baker's*), 1 oz. 140
bar, white (*Baker's*), 1 oz. 160
chips, all varieties (*Hershey's Bake Shoppe*), ½oz.,
1 tbsp. 80
chips, milk or semi-sweet (*Ghirardelli*), ½ oz., 1 tbsp. . . . 70
chips, white (*Ghirardelli*), ½ oz., 1 tbsp. 80
Chocolate drink:
bottled (Yoo Hoo), 9 fl. oz. 150
canned (Yoo Hoo), 11 fl. oz. 180
Chocolate flavor drink, canned:
canned, all flavors (*Sweet Success*), 10 fl. oz. 200
canned, creamy milk (*Nestlé Instant Breakfast*), 10 fl. oz. 220
refrigerated, all flavors (*Sweet Success*), 12 fl. oz. 220
Chocolate flavor drink mix:
(*Pillsbury* Instant Breakfast), 1 pkt. 140
all flavors (*Carnation Instant Breakfast*), 1 pkt. 130
all flavors (*Carnation Instant Breakfast* No Sugar), 1 pkt. . 70
all flavors (*Sweet Success*), 1.1 oz. 90
Chocolate milk:
(*Nestlé Quik*), 8 fl. oz. 230
lowfat (*Hershey's*), 8 fl. oz. 190
Chocolate pastry (*Pepperidge Farm* Clouds), 2 pieces . . 580
Chocolate syrup, regular or malt (*Hershey's*), 2 tbsp. . . 100
Chocolate topping, 2 tbsp:
all varieties (*Smucker's Magic Shell*) 220
caramel (*Hershey's*) 100
double or mint (*Hershey's*) 110
fudge, hot (*Hershey's*) 130
Chow chow pickle (*Crosse & Blackwell*), 1 tbsp. 10
Chow mein, see "Chicken entree" and "Beef entree"

Chrysanthemum garland, boiled, drained, 1″ pieces,
½ cup 10
Church's Chicken, 1 serving:
chicken, edible portion:
breast, 2.8 oz. 200
leg, 2 oz. 140
Tender Strip, 1.1 oz. 80
thigh, 2.8 oz. 230
wing, 3.1 oz. 250
sides:
biscuit, 2.1 oz. 250
Cajun rice, 3.1 oz. 130
coleslaw, 3 oz. 92
corn on cob, 5.7 oz. 139
french fries, 2.7 oz. 210
okra, 2.8 oz. 210
potatoes and gravy, 3.7 oz. 90
apple pie, 3.1 oz. 280
Churro, cinnamon (*Tio Pepe's*), 1-oz. piece 110
Chutney, 1 tbsp.:
mango (*Patak's* Major Grey's) 50
tomato, dried (*Sonoma*) 35
tropical fruit and nut (*Patak's*) 60
Cisco, meat only, raw, 4 oz. 112
Citron, candied:
(*S&W*), 39 pieces, 1.1 oz. 90
diced (*Paradise/White Swan*), 2 tbsp., .9 oz. 80
Citrus juice blend (*Pet/Season's Best* Medley), 8 fl. oz. 120
Citrus drink, 8 fl. oz.:
(*Five Alive*) 120
frozen*, (*Five Alive*) 110
punch (*Tropicana*) 140
punch, chilled or frozen* (*Minute Maid*) 120
punch, tropical, chilled or frozen* (*Five Alive*) 110
Clam, meat only, boiled, poached, or steamed, 4 oz. . . . 168
Clam, canned, ¼ cup or 2 oz.:
baby, whole (*S&W*) 50
chopped or minced (*Doxsee*) 25
chopped or minced (*S&W*) 20

Clam, canned ***(cont.)***
smoked (*S&W*) 130
Clam, frozen, fried (*Gorton's* Crunchy), 3 oz. 260
Clam dip, 2 tbsp.:
(*Breakstone's* Chesapeake) 50
(*Heluva* Good New England) 50
(*Nalley's*) 100
Clam entree, frozen, fried (*Mrs. Paul's*), 3 oz. 280
Clam juice (*S&W*), 9.6-fl. oz. can 20
Clam sauce, canned, ½ cup:
creamy (*Progresso*) 100
red (*Progresso*) 80
white (*Progresso*) 120
Clover seeds, sprouted, raw (*Shaw's*), 2 oz. 7
Clover sprouts (*Jonathan's*), 1 cup, 3 oz. 25
Cobbler, frozen:
apple (*Marie Callender's*), 4.25 oz. 350
berry or cherry (*Marie Callender's*), 4.25 oz. 390
blueberry (*Marie Callender's*), 4 oz. 340
peach (*Marie Callender's*), 4.25 oz. 370
Cocktail sauce, see "Seafood sauce"
Cocoa, unsweetened, 1 tbsp.:
(*Ghirardelli*) 35
(*Hershey's*) 20
(*Nestlé* Baking) 15
Cocoa mix, hot, 1 pkt., except as noted:
(*Carnation* Fat Free) 25
(*Carnation* No Sugar) 50
(*Swiss Miss/Swiss Miss* Premiere) 140
(*Swiss Miss* Diet) 20
(*Swiss Miss* Lite) 70
chocolate (*Swiss Miss* Sensations) 150
chocolate, double, hazelnut, or mocha (*Ghirardelli*) 90
chocolate, milk or rich (*Carnation*), 3 tbsp. 110
chocolate, milk, rich, white, or mini marshmallow (*Swiss Miss*) 110
chocolate, milk or mini marshmallow (*Swiss Miss* Sugar Free) 50
and cream (*Swiss Miss*) 150

Coconut, fresh, shelled, 1 oz. 100
Coconut, canned or packaged (*Angel Flake*), 2 tbsp. 70
Coconut cream, canned (*Coco Lopez*), 3 tbsp. 170
Coconut milk, canned:
(*Taste of Thai*), 1/4 cup 110
light (*Taste of Thai*), 1/4 cup 36
Coconut nectar (*R.W. Knudsen*), 8 fl. oz. 140
Cod, Atlantic or Pacific, baked, broiled, or microwaved, 4 oz. 119
Cod, canned, Atlantic, with liquid, 4 oz. 119
Cod, dried, Atlantic, salted, 1 oz. 81
Cod, frozen, Pacific, loins (*Peter Pan*), 4 oz. 90
Cod entree, breaded, frozen (*Mrs. Paul's*Premium), 1 fillet 240
Coffee, brewed, 6 fl. oz. 4
Coffee, flavored, see "Coffee, iced" and "Cappuccino"
Coffee, flavored, mix 8 fl. oz.*:
cafe Amaretto or Français (*General Foods International*) . 60
cafe Vienna (*General Foods International*) 70
cappuccino, Italian (*General Foods International*) 50
cappuccino, orange (*General Foods International*) 70
chocolate, Viennese (*General Foods International*) 60
hazelnut, Belgian (*General Foods International*) 70
mocha, Suisse (*General Foods International*) 60
vanilla, French (*General Foods International* Sugar Free) . 35
Coffee, iced (see also "Cappuccino"), canned, regular or latte (*Jamaican Gold*), 11-oz. can 140
Coffee creamer, see "Cream" and "Creamer, nondairy"
Coffee substitute, cereal grain (*Postum* Instant), 1 tsp. . 10
Cold cuts, see specific listings
Coleslaw, salad blend mix (*Dole*), 3.5 oz. 30
Collard greens:
fresh, boiled, drained, chopped, 1/2 cup 17
canned (*Allens/Sunshine*), 1/2 cup 30
frozen, chopped, boiled, drained, 1/2 cup 31
Cookie:
almond (*Archway* Crescents), 2 pieces, .8 oz. 100
almond (*Stella D'Oro* Chinese Dessert), 1.2-oz. piece . . . 170
almond (*Sunshine* Crescents), 4 pieces, 1.1 oz. 150

Cookie *(cont.)*

animal (*Sunshine*), 14 pieces, 1.1 oz. 140
anisette (*Stella D'Oro* Sponge), 2 pieces, 1 oz. 90
apple (*Newtons* Fat Free), 2 pieces, 1 oz. 100
apple and raisin (*Archway*), 1.1-oz. piece 130
(*Archway* Bells and Stars/Holiday Pac), 3 pieces, 1 oz. . . 150
(*Archway* Old Fashion Windmill), .75-oz. piece 100
(*Archway* Party Treats), 3 pieces, 1.1 oz. 140
(*Archway* Select Assortment), 4 pieces, 1.1 oz. 160
biscotti, all varieties (*Health Valley*), 2 pieces 120
biscottini cashews (*Stella D'Oro*), .7-oz. piece 110
butter (*Peek Freans* Petit Beurre), 4 pieces, 1 oz. 130
butter (*Sunshine*), 5 pieces, 1.1 oz. 140
chocolate fudge (*Dare*), .7-oz. piece 97
chocolate fudge mint (*Grasshopper*), 4 pieces, 1.1 oz. . . 150
chocolate wafer (*Nabisco* Famous), 5 pieces, 1.1 oz. . . . 140
chocolate chip or chunk:
(*Archway*), 1-oz. piece 130
(*Archway* Drop/Ice Box/Toffee), 1-oz. piece 140
(*Chip-A-Roos*), 3 pieces, 1.3 oz. 190
(*Chips Ahoy!* Chewy), 3 pieces, 1.3 oz. 170
(*Chips Ahoy!* Chunky/Striped), .6-oz. piece 80
(*Chips Ahoy!* Real Chocolate), 3 pieces, 1.1 oz. 160
(*Chips Ahoy!* Reduced Fat), 3 pieces, 1.1 oz. 150
(*Chips Deluxe*), .5-oz. piece 80
(*Chips Deluxe* Chocolate Lovers), .6-oz. piece 90
(*Chips Deluxe* Light), .6-oz. piece 70
(*Grandma's* Big), 1.4-oz. piece 190
(*Pepperidge Farm* Old Fashioned), 3 pieces, 1 oz. . . . 140
(*Snackwell's* Reduced Fat), 13 pieces, 1 oz. 130
all varieties (*Health Valley Healthy Chips* Fat Free),
3 pieces 100
fudge (*Grandma's* Big), 1.4-oz. piece 170
macadamia, soft (*Pepperidge Farm*), .9-oz. piece . . . 130
mini (*Sunshine*), 5 pieces, 1.1 oz. 160
snaps (*Nabisco*), 7 pieces, 1.1 oz. 150
soft (*Chips Deluxe*), 1 piece, .5 oz. 70
soft (*Pepperidge Farm* Chocolate Walnut/Chunk),
.9-oz. piece 130

sprinkled (*Chips Ahoy!*), 3 pieces, 1.3 oz. 170
chocolate sandwich (*Hydrox*), 3 pieces, 1.1 oz. 150
chocolate sandwich (*Oreo*), 3 pieces, 1.2 oz. 160
chocolate sandwich (*Snackwell's* Reduced Fat), 2 pieces, .9 oz. 100
cinnamon apple (*Archway*), 1-oz. piece 110
cocoa, Dutch (*Archway*), 1-oz. piece 120
coconut (*Dare Breaktime*), .3-oz. piece 35
coconut, macaroon (*Archway*), .8-oz. piece 90
cranberry (*Newtons* Fat Free), 2 pieces, 1 oz. 100
Danish (*Nabisco* Import), 5 pieces, 1.2 oz. 170
devil's food cake (*Snackwell's* Fat Free), .6-oz. piece 50
egg biscuit, Roman (*Stella D'Oro*), 1.2 oz. piece 140
fig (*Fig Newtons*), 2 pieces, 1.1 oz. 110
fig (*Fig Newtons* Fat Free), 2 pieces, 1 oz. 100
fortune (*La Choy*), 4 pieces, 1.1 oz. 110
fruit and honey bar (*Archway*), 1-oz. piece 110
fudge (*Stella D'Oro* Swiss), 2 pieces, .9 oz. 130
fudge mint patties (*Sunshine*), 2 pieces, .8 oz. 130
fudge nut bar (*Archway*), 1-oz. piece 110
ginger (*Dare Breaktime*), .3-oz. piece 34
ginger snaps (*Archway*), 5 pieces, 1.1 oz. 140
ginger snaps (*Nabisco* Old Fashion), 4 pieces, 1 oz. . . . 120
ginger snaps (*Sunshine*), 7 pieces, 1 oz. 130
gingerbread, iced (*Archway*), 3 pieces, 1.1 oz. 140
gingerbread, iced (*Sunshine*), 5 pieces, 1 oz. 130
graham (*Nabisco*), 8 pieces, 1 oz. 120
graham, cinnamon (*Honey Maid*), 10 pieces, 1.1 oz. . . . 140
graham, cinnamon, snacks (*Snackwell's* Fat Free), 20 pieces, 1.1 oz. 110
graham, honey (*Honey Maid*), 8 pieces, 1 oz. 120
hermits (*Archway* Cookie Jar), 1-oz. piece 110
(*Heyday*), ¾-oz. bar 110
lemon (*Sunshine* Coolers), 5 pieces, 1.1 oz. 140
lemon, frosty (*Archway*), 1-oz. piece 120
marshmallow, chocolate (*Mallomars*), 2 pieces, .9 oz. . . 120
marshmallow, chocolate (*Pinwheels*), 1.1-oz. piece 130
mint sandwich (*Mystic Mint*), .6-oz. piece 90
molasses (*Archway* Old Fashion), 1-oz. piece 120

Cookie *(cont.)*

mud pie (*Archway*), 1-oz. piece 110
New Orleans cake (*Archway*), 1-oz. piece 110
nut (*Archway* Nutty Nougat), 3 pieces, 1.1 oz. 160
nut (*Little Debbie Nutty Bars*), 2 pieces, 1.2 oz. 180
oatmeal (*Archway*), 1-oz. piece 110
oatmeal (*Dare Breaktime*), .3-oz. piece 35
oatmeal (*Nabisco* Family Favorites), .6-oz. piece 80
oatmeal (*Sunshine* Country), 3 pieces, 1.2 oz. 170
oatmeal, apple or date filled (*Archway*), 1-oz. piece 110
oatmeal, iced or pecan (*Archway*), 1-oz. piece 120
oatmeal, iced (*Sunshine*), 2 pieces, .9 oz. 120
oatmeal raisin (*Archway*), 1-oz. piece 110
oatmeal raisin (*Little Debbie*), 2 pieces, 1.3 oz. 170
oatmeal raisin (*Snackwell's* Reduced Fat), 2 pieces, 1 oz. 110
peanut crunch (*Archway*), 6 pieces, 1.1 oz. 150
peanut butter (*Archway*), 1-oz. piece 140
peanut butter sandwich (*Nutter Butter*), 2 pieces, 1 oz. . . 130
pecan (*Archway* Ice Box), 1-oz. piece 140
raisin (*Dare Sun-Maid*), .5-oz. piece 52
raspberry (*Newtons* Fat Free), 2 pieces, 1 oz. 100
sesame (*Stella D'Oro* Regina), 3 pieces, 1.1 oz. 150
shortbread (*Lorna Doone*), 4 pieces, 1 oz. 140
shortbread (*Simply Sandies*), .5-oz. piece 80
shortbread, butter (*Dare*), .5-oz. piece 63
shortbread, fudge striped (*Sunshine*), 3 pieces, 1.1 oz. . . 160
shortbread, pecan (*Pecan Sandies*), .6-oz. piece 80
(*Social Tea*), 6 pieces, 1 oz. 120
spice, pfeffernusse (*Archway*), 2 pieces, 1.3 oz. 140
(*Stella D'Oro Angelica Goodies*), .8-oz. piece 100
(*Stella D'Oro Angel Wings*), 2 pieces, .9 oz. 140
(*Stella D'Oro Anginetti*), 4 pieces, 1.1 oz. 140
(*Stella D'Oro Como Delights*), 1.1 oz. 140
strawberry (*Newtons* Fat Free), 2 pieces, 1 oz. 100
sugar (*Archway*), 1-oz. piece 120
sugar (*Dare*), .3-oz. piece 39
sugar wafer, chocolate (*Sunshine*), 3 pieces, .9 oz. 130
sugar wafer, peanut butter (*Sunshine*), 4 pieces, 1.1 oz. 170
sugar wafer, vanilla (*Sunshine*), 3 pieces, .9 oz. 130

vanilla (*Stella D'Oro* Margherite), 2 pieces, 1.1 oz. 140
vanilla sandwich (*Cameo*), 2 pieces 130
vanilla sandwich (*Cookie Break*), 3 pieces 160
vanilla sandwich (*Snackwell's* Reduced Fat), 2 pieces, .9 oz. 110
vanilla sandwich (*Vienna Fingers*), 2 pieces 130
vanilla wafer (*Nilla*), 8 pieces, 1.1 oz. 140
vanilla wafer (*Sunshine*), 7 pieces, 1.1 oz. 150
vanilla sandwich (*Cameo*), 2 pieces, 1 oz. 130
vanilla sandwich (*Nabisco* Family Favorites), 3 pieces, 1.2 oz. 170
vanilla sandwich (*Vienna Fingers*), 2 pieces, 1 oz. 130
walnut, black (*Archway* Ice Box), .8-oz. piece 120

Cookie, refrigerated:

chocolate chip (*Pillsbury*), 1 oz. 130
chocolate chip, oatmeal (*Pillsbury*), 1 oz. 120
chocolate chocolate chip (*Pillsbury*), 1 oz. 130
peanut butter (*Pillsbury*), 1 oz. 110
sugar (*Pillsbury*), 2 pieces 130

Cookie bar mix:

(*Betty Crocker Easy Layer Bars*), 1/20 pkg. 120
apple cinnamon or banana (*Sweet Rewards*), 1/8 pkg. . . . 170
apple streusel bar (*Pillsbury*), 1 bar* 150
chocolate (*Sweet Rewards*), 1/8 pkg. 160
chocolate chip bar (*Pillsbury Chips Ahoy!*), 1 bar* 180
chocolate chunk bar (*Betty Crocker*), 1/32 pkg. 80
chocolate cookie bar (*Pillsbury Oreo*), 1 bar* 150
chocolate peanut butter bar (*Betty Crocker*), 1/12 pkg. . . . 170
date bar (*Betty Crocker*), 1/12 pkg.* 150
fudge swirl cookie (*Pillsbury*), 1 bar* 180
gingerbread (*Betty Crocker*), 1/8 pkg. 220
lemon (*Sweet Rewards*), 1/8 pkg. 170
lemon bar (*Betty Crocker Sunkist*), 1/16 pkg. 130
lemon cheesecake bar (*Pillsbury*), 1 bar* 180
peanut butter bar (*Pillsbury Nutter Butter*), 1 bar* 180
raspberry (*Betty Crocker*), 1/20 pkg. 150

Corn, 1/2 cup, except as noted:

fresh, kernels, boiled, drained 89
canned, baby (*Roland*) 25

Corn ***(cont.)***

canned, kernel (*S&W* Sweet 'n Crisp), 1/3 cup 70
canned, kernel, regular or white (*Stokely/Stokely* No Salt) . 90
canned, kernel, with peppers (*Stokely*), 1/3 cup 80
canned, cream style (*S&W*) 100
canned, cream style, regular or white (*Stokely*) 100
frozen, on the cob (*John Cope's*) 1 ear 120
frozen, on the cob, white (*John Cope's*) 1 ear 150
frozen, kernel (*Green Giant Niblets*), 2/3 cup 80
frozen, kernel, white (*John Cope's*), 1/3 cup 80
frozen, cream style (*Green Giant*) 110
frozen, cream style, white (*John Cope's* Sweet 'N Creamy), 1/3 cup 100
in butter sauce (*Green Giant Niblets*), 2/3 cup 130

Corn chips, puffs, and similar snacks, 1 oz., except as noted:

(*Barrel O'Fun* Chips), 1.1 oz. 160
(*Bugles*), 1 1/3 cups 160
(*Bugles* Light), 1 1/2 cups 130
(*Fritos* King Size/Original/Wild N' Mild) 160
(*Fritos* Scoops) 150
(*Old Dutch* Chips), 1.1 oz. 170
(*Old Dutch Puffcorn* Curls), 1.1 oz. 180
(*Planters* Chips) 160
(*Sunchips* Original) 140
all varieties (*Santitas* Chips/Crisps/100%) 140
barbecue (*Fritos*) 150
barbecue (*Old Dutch*), 1.1 oz. 165
cheese (*Chee·tos* Cheesy Checkers/Crunchy) 150
cheese, all varieties (*Combos*) 140
cheese, cheddar (*Sunchips* Harvest) 140
cheese, hot (*Chee·tos* Flamin') 160
cheese balls (*Chee·tos*) 150
cheese balls or curls (*Planters* Cheez) 150
cheese puffs (*Chee·tos*) 160
chili cheese (*Fritos*) 160
tortilla (*No Fries* Natural) 100
tortilla (*Old Dutch* Restaurant) 140
tortilla (*Santitas* Chips/Strips) 140

tortilla (*Tostitos* Baked/Baked Unsalted) 110
tortilla (*Tostitos* Crispy Round) 150
tortilla (*Tostitos* Restaurant/Santa Fe Gold/Unsalted) . . . 140
tortilla (*Tyson* Yellow Corn), 1.1 oz. 150
tortilla, all varieties (*Doritos*) 140
tortilla, all varieties (*Doritos* Reduced Fat) 130
tortilla, blue cheese (*Barbara's* Pinta Blues) 130
tortilla, lime and chili (*Kettle* Tias) 140
tortilla, lime and chili (*Tostitos*) 150
tortilla, nacho cheese (*Old Dutch*), 1-oz. bag 140
tortilla, nacho cheese (*Tyson*) 140
Corn flake crumbs (*Kellogg's*), 2 tbsp. 40
Corn flour (see also "Cornmeal"):
whole grain, 1 cup 422
masa, 1 cup 416
Corn fritter, frozen (*Mrs. Paul's*), 1 piece 130
Corn grits, dry:
instant, all varieties, except with ham bits (*Quaker*),
1-oz. pkt. 100
instant, with ham bits (*Quaker*), 1-oz. pkt. 90
white (*Quaker* Hominy), 1/4 cup 140
white (*Quaker* Quick Hominy), 1/4 cup 130
yellow (*Quaker* Quick Hominy), 1/4 cup 120
Corn relish (*Nance's*), 2 tbsp. 25
Corn syrup, dark or light (*Karo*), 2 tbsp. 120
Cornish hen:
cooked, dark meat (*Perdue*), 3 oz. 200
cooked, white meat (*Perdue*), 3 oz. 170
half, roasted, dark meat (*Perdue*), 6.5 oz. 210
half, roasted, white meat (*Perdue*), 6.5 oz. 200
Cornmeal (see also "Polenta"):
blue or hi-lysine (*Arrowhead Mills*), 1/4 cup 130
blue and red (*Frieda's*), 1/2 cup 214
self-rising, buttermilk, regular or white (*Aunt Jemima*
Mix), 3 tbsp. 80
self-rising, yellow (*Aunt Jemima* Mix), 3 tbsp. 90
Cornstarch (*Argo/Kingsford*), 1 tbsp. 30
Country gravy mix (*Durkee/French's*), 1/4 cup* 35

Couscous:
dry, (*Fantastic Foods*), 1/4 cup 210
dry, whole wheat (*Fantastic Foods*), 1/4 cup 180
cooked, 1/2 cup 101
Couscous mix, 1 container, except as noted:
almond chicken, vegetarian (*Casbah*) 160
asparagus au gratin (*Casbah*) 150
black bean salsa (*Fantastic* Cup) 240
cheddar, broccoli, creamy (*Casbah*) 130
cheddar, nacho (*Fantastic* Cup) 200
corn, sweet (*Fantastic* Cup) 180
with lentils (*Fantastic Only A Pinch* Cup) 220
pilaf (*Casbah*), 1 oz. 100
savory pilaf (*Fantastic Foods*), 1 cup 240
tomato Parmesan (*Casbah*) 170
vegetable, Creole (*Fantastic* Cup) 220
Cowpeas:
fresh, boiled, drained, 1/2 cup 79
fresh, leafy tips, boiled, drained, 4 oz. 25
fresh, pods with seeds, boiled, drained, 1/2 cup 16
fresh, mature, boiled, 1/2 cup 100
frozen, boiled, drained, 1/2 cup 112
canned, see "Black-eyed peas"
Crab, meat only, 4 oz., except as noted:
Alaska king, boiled, poached, or steamed 110
blue, boiled, poached, or steamed 116
Dungeness, boiled, poached, or steamed 125
queen, boiled, poached, or steamed 130
Crab, canned, Dungeness (*S&W*), 1/3 cup, 3 oz. 80
"Crab," imitation, frozen or refrigerated:
(*Peter Pan*), 3 oz. 70
chunk or leg style (*Louis Kemp Crab Delights*), 3 oz.,
3 legs 80
flaked (*Seafest*), 1/2 cup, 3 oz. 100
Crab cake, deviled, frozen:
(*Mrs. Paul's*), 3-oz. cake 170
miniature (*Mrs. Paul's*), 6 pieces, 3.5 oz. 230
Crabapple:
fresh, with peel, sliced, 1/2 cup 42

canned (*S&W*), 1 piece 35
canned, spiced (*Apple Time*), 1.1-oz. apple 40

Cracker:

assorted (*Pepperidge Farm*), 3 pieces, ½ oz. 60
butter or butter flavor:
 (*Hi-Ho*), 9 pieces, 1.1 oz. 160
 (*Keebler Club* Partners), 4 pieces, ½ oz. 70
 (*Ritz/Ritz* Low Sodium), 5 pieces, .6 oz. 80
 (*Toasted Complements* Buttercrisp), 9 pieces, 1 oz. . . 140
 (*Town House*), 5 pieces, .6 oz. 80
 mini (*Ritz Bits*), 48 pieces, 1.1 oz. 160
cheese (*Nips*), 29 pieces, 1.1 oz. 150
cheese (*Snackwell's*), 38 pieces, 1.1 oz. 130
cheese (*Tid-Bit*), 32 pieces, 1.1 oz. 150
cheese, all varieties (*Appeteasers*), 1 oz. 130
cheese, cheddar (*Better Cheddars*), 22 pieces, 1.1 oz. . . 150
cheese, cheddar (*Better Cheddars* Reduced Fat),
 24 pieces, 1.1 oz. 140
cheese, cheddar (*Cheez-It/Cheez-It* Low Sodium),
 27 pieces, 1.1 oz. 160
cheese, cheddar (*Cheez-It* Reduced Fat), 30 pieces,
 1.1 oz. 130
cheese, zesty (*Snackwell's*), 32 pieces, 1.1 oz. 120
cheese sandwich:
 (*Ritz*), 1.4-oz. pkg. 210
 (*Ritz Bits*), 14 pieces, 1.1 oz. 160
 bacon or wheat (*Frito-Lay*), 1 pkg. 200
 cheddar, golden toast (*Frito-Lay*), 1 pkg. 230
 cheddar, jalapeño (*Frito-Lay*), 1 pkg. 200
 cream cheese and chive, golden toast (*Frito-Lay*),
 1 pkg. 240
chicken flavor (*Chicken In A Biskit*), 14 pieces, 1.1 oz. . . 160
croissant (*Carr's*), 3 pieces, ½ oz. 70
flatbread, 8 pieces, 1 oz., except as noted:
 all varieties (*J.J. Flats*), ½-oz. piece 50
 caraway rye or peppercorn (*Lavosh Hawaii*) 115
 onion or plain (*Lavosh Hawaii* Classic) 120
 rosemary garlic (*Lavosh Hawaii*) 125
 10 grain (*Lavosh Hawaii*) 110

Cracker ***(cont.)***

golden (*Snackwell's* Classic), 6 pieces, ½ oz. 60
graham, see "Cookie"
matzo (*Manischewitz* Unsalted/Everything!), 1 oz. 110
matzo, garlic (*Manischewitz* Savory), 1 oz. 100
matzo, rye (*Manischewitz*), 1 oz. 110
melba rounds, all varieties (*Old London*), 5 pieces, ½ oz. . 60
melba toast, all varieties except whole grain (*Old London*), ½ oz. 50
melba toast, whole grain (*Old London*), 3 pieces, ½ oz. . 45
milk (*Royal Lunch*), .4-oz. piece 50
multigrain (*Hi-Ho*), 9 pieces, 1.1 oz. 160
multigrain (*Wheat Thins*), 17 pieces, 1.1 oz. 130
oat (*Oat Thins*), 18 pieces, 1.1 oz. 140
onion (*Toasted Complements*), 9 pieces, 1 oz. 140
onion, French (*Snackwell's*), 32 pieces, 1.1 oz. 120
onion, French (*Wheatables*), 27 pieces, 1.1 oz. 130
peanut butter sandwich (*Ritz*), 13 pieces, 1.1 oz. 150
peanut butter sandwich, cheese or toast (*Planters*), 1.4-oz. pkg. 190
potato, all varieties (*No Fries*), 1.1 oz. 110
ranch (*Munch'ems*), 33 pieces, 1.1 oz. 130
salsa (*Munch'ems*), 28 pieces, 1.1 oz. 130
saltines, all varieties (*Krispy*), 5 pieces, ½ oz. 60
sesame (*Breton*), 10 pieces, 1.5 oz. 220
sesame (*Toasted Complements*), 9 pieces, 1 oz. 140
sour cream and onion (*Munch'ems*), 33 pieces, 1.1 oz. 130
soup and oyster (*Oysterettes/Premium*), ½ oz. 60
10 grain (*Lavosh Hawaii*) 110
water or soda:
(*Breton/Breton* Less Salt), 10 pieces, 1.5 oz. 210
(*Breton* Light), 10 pieces, 1.5 oz. 200
(*Cabaret*), 10 pieces, 1.7 oz. 230
(*Hi-Ho*), 9 pieces, 1.1 oz. 160
(*Vivant*), 10 pieces, 1.5 oz. 210
cracked pepper (*Hi-Ho*), 9 pieces, 1.1 oz. 160
sesame (*Breton*), 10 pieces, 1.5 oz. 220
wheat (*Snackwell's* Fat Free), 5 pieces, ½ oz. 60
wheat (*Stoned Wheat Thins*), 2 pieces 60

wheat (*Toasted Complements*), 9 pieces, 1 oz. 140
wheat (*Triscuit*), 7 pieces, 1.1 oz. 140
wheat (*Waverly*), 5 pieces, ½ oz. 70
wheat (*Wheat Thins/Wheat Thins* Low Salt), 16 pieces, 1 oz. 140
wheat, garden herb (*Triscuit*), 6 pieces, 1 oz. 130
wheat, and rye (*Triscuit* Deli-Style), 7 pieces, 1.1 oz. . . . 140
wheat, whole (*Carr's*), 2 pieces, .6 oz. 80
wheat, whole (*Hi-Ho*), 9 pieces, 1.1 oz. 150
wheat, whole, and bran (*Triscuit*), 7 pieces, 1.1 oz. 140
(*Zwieback*), .3-oz. piece 35

Cracker crumbs and meal:
crumbs, saltine (*Premium* Fat Free), ¼ cup 100
matzo meal (*Manischewitz*), ¼ cup 130

Cranberry, fresh, raw, whole, ½ cup 23
Cranberry, dried (*Sonoma*), ⅓ cup 120
Cranberry bean, boiled, ½ cup 120
Cranberry drink, 8 fl. oz.:
(*Tropicana* Punch) 140
(*Tropicana* Ruby Red) 120

Cranberry drink blends, 8 fl. oz.:
hibiscus (*Heinke's/R.W. Knudsen*) 120
lemon (*Santa Cruz*) 120
raspberry (*R.W. Knudsen*) 140

Cranberry juice, 8 fl. oz.:
(*After the Fall* Cape Cod) 100
(*Apple & Eve Naturally Cranberry*) 120
(*Snapple* Royal), 10 fl. oz. 150

Cranberry juice blend:
grape (*Apple & Eve*), 10 fl. oz. 175
grapefruit, mango, or orange (*After the Fall*), 8 fl. oz. . . . 110
kiwi or strawberry (*After the Fall*), 8 fl. oz. 100

Cranberry nectar, plain or guava (*Santa Cruz*), 8 fl. oz. 110
Cranberry sauce, canned, whole or jellied (*S&W*), ¼ cup 100
Cranberry-orange relish, in jars (*New England*), ¼ cup 120
Crayfish, meat only, wild or farmed, boiled or steamed, 4 oz. 100
Cream (see also "Cream, sour" and "Creamer, nondairy"):

Cream ***(cont.)***
half and half, 1 tbsp. 20
light, coffee or table, 1 tbsp. .29
medium (25% fat), 1 tbsp. 37
whipping, light, 1 tbsp. (2 tbsp. whipped) 44
whipping, heavy, 1 tbsp. (2 tbsp. whipped) 52
whipped topping, see "Cream topping"
Cream, canned, light (*Nestlé* Crema), 1 tbsp. 30
Cream, sour, 2 tbsp.:
(*Heluva* Good) 60
light (*Heluva* Good) 40
nondairy, plain or flavored (*Sour Supreme*) 50
nonfat (*Heluva* Good) 20
Cream topping, 2 tbsp.:
(*Cool Whip* Extra Creamy) 30
(*Cool Whip* Lite) 20
(*Cool Whip* Nondairy) 25
pressurized can (*Rich's*) .25
Cream topping, mix* (*Dream Whip*) 2 tbsp. 20
Creamer, nondairy, 1 tbsp., except as noted:
(*Rich's Coffee Rich*) 25
(*Rich's Coffee Rich* Light) 15
(*Rich's Farm Rich*) 20
(*Rich's Farm Rich* Light/Fat Free) 10
liquid (*Coffee-mate*) 20
liquid, lite (*Coffee-mate* Fat Free/Lite) 10
powder, all varieties (*Coffee-mate*), 1 tsp. 10
Cress, garden, raw, ½ cup .8
Cress, water, see "Watercress"
Croissant:
butter (*Awrey's*), 2-oz. piece 190
butter (*Pepperidge Farm* Petite), 1 piece 130
frozen (*Sara Lee*), 1 piece 170
Crookneck squash:
fresh, boiled, drained, sliced, ½ cup 18
canned, cut, drained, ½ cup 14
Croutons, ¼ oz. or 2 tbsp.:
all varieties (*Arnold* Crispy/*Brownberry*) 30
all varieties (*Old London* Restaurant Style) 30

Cucumber, with peel, sliced, ½ cup 7
Cucumber salad (*Rosoff/Schorr's*), 1 oz. 12
Currants:
fresh, trimmed, black, European, ½ cup 36
fresh, trimmed, red or white, ½ cup 31
dried, zante (*S&W*), ¼ cup 130
Curry paste (*Patak's*), 2 tbsp. 170
Curry powder, 1 tbsp. 20
Curry sauce, cooking:
(*Kylin Thai*), ¼ cup 25
Jalfrezzi (*Patak's*), ½ cup 160
Madras, hot (*Patak's*), ½ cup 300
Masala (*Shahi* Cream/Curry), ¼ cup 50
Rogan Josh (*Patak's*), ½ cup 190
tikka Masala (*Patak's*), ½ cup 240
vindaloo, hot (*Patak's*), ½ cup 320
Custard, see "Pudding mix"
Custard apple, trimmed, 1 oz. 29
Cuttlefish, meat only, boiled or steamed, 4 oz. 179
Cuttlefish, canned, in ink (*Goya*), ¼ cup 120

D

FOOD AND MEASURE	CALORIES
Daikon, see "Radish, Oriental"	
Daiquiri mixer:	
bottled (*Holland House*), 4 fl. oz.	150
frozen*, strawberry (*Bacardi*), 8 fl. oz.	140
Dairy Queen/Brazier, 1 serving:	
DQ Homestyle burgers:	
cheeseburger	340
cheeseburger, deluxe double	540
cheeseburger with bacon, double	610
hamburger	290
hamburger, deluxe double	440
Ultimate burger	670
sandwiches:	
chicken fillet, breaded	430
chicken fillet, breaded with cheese	480
chicken fillet, grilled	310
fish fillet	370
fish fillet with cheese	420
hot dog	240
hot dog with cheese	290
hot dog with chili	280
hot dog with chili and cheese	330
chicken strip basket, with gravy	860
chicken strip basket, with BBQ sauce	810
side dishes:	
french fries, large	390
french fries, regular	300
french fries, small	210
onion rings, regular	240
desserts and shakes:	
banana split	510
Blizzard, Butterfinger, regular	750
Blizzard, chocolate chip cookie dough, regular	950

Blizzard, chocolate sandwich cookie, regular 640
Blizzard, Heath, regular 820
Blizzard, Reese's peanut butter cup, regular 790
Blizzard, strawberry, regular 570
Buster Bar 450
cone, chocolate, regular 360
cone, chocolate-dipped, regular 510
cone, vanilla, regular 350
DQ caramel and nut bar 260
DQ fudge bar 50
DQ Lemon Freez'r, ½ cup 80
DQ sandwich 150
DQ Treatzza Pizza, Heath, or strawberry-banana,
⅛ pie 180
DQ Treatzza Pizza, M&M, ⅛ pie 190
DQ Treatzza Pizza, peanut butter fudge, ⅛ pie 220
DQ vanilla orange bar 60
Dilly bar, chocolate 210
Dilly bar, chocolate mint 190
Dilly bar, toffee, w/*Heath* pieces 210
Fudge Nut Bar 410
malt, chocolate, regular 880
Misty cooler, strawberry 190
Misty slush, regular 290
Peanut Buster parfait 730
Queen's Choice Big Scoop, chocolate 250
Queen's Choice Big Scoop, vanilla 250
shake, chocolate, regular 770
soft serve, *DQ* chocolate, ½ cup 150
soft serve, *DQ* vanilla, ½ cup 140
Starkiss 80
strawberry shortcake 430
sundae, chocolate, regular 410
yogurt, frozen, *Breeze, Heath,* regular 710
yogurt, frozen, *Breeze,* strawberry, regular 460
yogurt, frozen, *DQ* Nonfat, ½ cup 100
yogurt, frozen, regular cup 230
yogurt, frozen, cone 280
yogurt, frozen, strawberry sundae 300

Dandelion greens, fresh, boiled, drained, chopped, 1/2 cup 17
Danish, 1 pastry:
all varieties (*Awrey's* Petite), 1.5 oz. 130
apple (*Hostess* Fruit Roll), 2 oz. 180
apple, cheese, or strawberry (*Awrey's*), 2 3/4 oz. 300
cheese, cherry (*Awrey's* Marquise), 3 1/4 oz. 350
cheese, lemon (*Awrey's* Marquise), 3 1/4 oz. 350
cinnamon swirl (*Awrey's*), 2 3/4 oz. 300
Danish, frozen or refrigerated, 1 piece:
apple or raspberry (*Pepperidge Farm*) 210
cheese (*Pepperidge Farm*) 230
Date:
dehydrated, coarse ground (*Dole*), 1 oz. 110
dried, whole, pitted, (*Dole*), 1/2 cup 280
dried, chopped, (*Dole*), 1/2 cup 230
Date nut pastry (*Awrey's*), 1.2 oz. 130
Dessert mix, chilled, no-bake, dry:
banana cream (*Betty Crocker*), 1/9 pkg. 160
chocolate French silk (*Betty Crocker*), 1/8 pkg. 180
coconut cream (*Betty Crocker*), 1/9 pkg. 200
cookies 'n creme (*Betty Crocker*) 1/6 pkg. 260
lemon supreme (*Betty Crocker*), 1/9 pkg. 270
Dill, weed, fresh, 1/2 cup loosely packed 2
Dill dip, 2 tbsp.:
pickle (*Nalley's*) 70
sour cream (*Marie's*) 190
vegetable, zesty (*Bernstein's*) 120
Dolphinfish, meat only, baked, broiled, or microwaved, 4 oz. 124
Donut, 1 piece:
plain (*Awrey's*), 2 oz. 240
plain (*Hostess* Old Fashioned), 1.5 oz. 170
chocolate iced (*Awrey's*), 1.75 oz. 200
chocolate iced (*Hostess*), 1.4 oz. 180
chocolate iced, chocolate (*Awrey's*), 1.75 oz. 190
chocolate iced, custard Bismark (*Awrey's*), 1 piece 350
cinnamon (*Hostess*), 1 oz. 110
coconut topped (*Awrey's*), 1.75 oz. 210

crunch (*Awrey's*), 2.5 oz. 280
crunch topped (*Awrey's*), 1.75 oz. 160
glazed (*Hostess* Old Fashioned), 2.2 oz. 250
glazed, honey, devil's food (*Awrey's*), 1 piece 310
powdered sugar (*Awrey's*), 1.5 oz. 170
powdered sugar (*Hostess*), 1 oz. 110
powdered sugar or vanilla iced, jelly Bismark (*Awrey's*),
3 oz. 320
sprinkle topped (*Awrey's*), 1.5 oz. 160
vanilla iced (*Awrey's* Long John), 3.4 oz. 380
white, iced (*Awrey's*), 1.75 oz. 200
Donut, frozen, glazed (*Rich's*), 1 cake 130
Duck, domesticated:
meat with skin, roasted, 4 oz. 382
meat only, roasted, 4 oz. 228
Duck sauce, see "Sweet and sour sauce"

E

FOOD AND MEASURE	CALORIES
Eclair, chocolate, frozen (*Rich's*), 1 piece	190
Eel, meat only, baked, broiled, or microwaved, 4 oz.	268
Egg, chicken:	
raw, whole, 1 large	75
raw, white only, from 1 large egg	17
raw, yolk only (with small portion white), from 1 large egg	59
cooked, hard-boiled, chopped, 1 cup	210
Egg, substitute or imitation, ¼ cup:	
(*Egg Beaters*)	30
(*Second Nature*)	40
Egg breakfast, frozen, 1 pkg.:	
patty, egg, with Canadian bacon (*Swanson Great Starts*)	240
patty, egg, with pork and turkey (*Swanson Great Starts*)	280
scrambled (*Swanson Great Starts* Egg Product)	240
scrambled, and bacon (*Swanson Great Starts*)	290
scrambled, with home fries (*Swanson Great Starts*)	200
scrambled, and sausage (*Swanson Great Starts*)	360
Egg breakfast sandwich, frozen, 1 piece or pkg.:	
with cheese (*Swanson Great Starts*)	360
muffin, with bacon and cheese (*Swanson Great Starts*)	290
muffin, with Canadian bacon, cheese (*Hormel Quick Meal*)	260
muffin, with sausage and cheese (*Hormel Quick Meal*)	390
Egg roll, frozen:	
(*Empire* Kosher), 3-oz. roll	190
chicken or pork (*La Choy*), 3-oz. roll	170
chicken or pork and shrimp mini (*La Choy*), 14 rolls, 7.25 oz.	430
chicken, sweet and sour (*La Choy*), 3-oz. roll	180
mini (*Empire* Kosher), 6 rolls, 4.9 oz.	280
pork, moo shu (*La Choy*), 3-oz. roll	190
shrimp (*La Choy*), 3-oz. roll	150

shrimp, mini (*La Choy*), 14 rolls, 7.25 oz. 410
vegetables with lobster, mini (*La Choy*), 14 rolls, 7.25 oz. 410
Egg roll wrapper (*Frieda's*), 2 pieces, 1.7 oz. 132
Eggnog, dairy (*Crowley*), ½ cup 190
Eggplant, fresh:
raw, trimmed, 1″ pieces, ½ cup 11
boiled, drained, 1″ cubes, ½ cup 13
Japanese, raw, with peel (*Frieda's*), 3.5 oz. 25
Eggplant appetizer, in jars:
roasted (*Peloponnese*), 2 tbsp. 25
stuffed, baby (*Krinos*), 1.1 oz., about 2 pieces 20
stuffed, rolettes (*Paesana*), 3.75 oz. 260
Eggplant entree, frozen:
cutlets (*Celentano*), 5 oz. 210
parmigiana (*Celentano*), 10-oz. pkg. 420
parmigiana (*Celentano* 14 oz.), ½ pkg. 320
parmigiana (*Celentano* Value Pack), 1 cup, 8 oz. 360
parmigiana (*Mrs. Paul's*), ½ cup 220
rollettes (*Celentano*), 10 oz. 350
rollettes (*Celentano* Great Choice), 10 oz. 330
Eggplant pickle (*Patak's* Brinjal Relish), 1 tbsp. 60
Elderberries, fresh, ½ cup 53
Empanadilla, frozen:
plain (*Goya*), 2 pieces 380
plain, cocktail (*Goya*), 7 pieces 370
Enchilada, canned (*Gebhardt*), 2 pieces 260
Enchilada dinner, frozen:
(*Amy's*), 10 oz. 250
(*Chi-Chi's* Baja), 15.4 oz. 580
(*Chi-Chi's* Chix Suprema), 14.9 oz. 580
beef (*Patio*), 12 oz. 350
beef or beef and cheese (*Patio* Chili 'n Beans Large), 2 pieces 250
cheese (*Patio*), 12 oz. 330
chicken (*Patio*), 12 oz. 380
Enchilada entree, frozen:
beef (*Banquet*), 11 oz. 380
beef (*Patio* Family Pack), 2 pieces 200

Enchilada entree *(cont.)*
beef and tamale, chili gravy with (*Morton*), 10 oz. 260
black bean (*Amy's* Family Size), 4.38 oz. 120
black bean, and vegetable (*Amy's* Family Size), 4.75 oz. 130
cheese (*Amy's*), 4.75 oz. 210
cheese (*Banquet*), 11 oz. 340
cheese (*Patio* Family Pack), 2 pieces 170
cheese, and rice (*Stouffer's*), 9¾ oz. 370
chicken (*Banquet*), 11 oz. 360
chicken, nacho grande (*Weight Watchers*), 9 oz. 290
chicken, and rice (*Stouffer's*), 9¾ oz. 370
chicken Suiza (*Healthy Choice*), 10 oz. 270
chicken Suiza (*Weight Watchers*), 9 oz. 270
chicken Suiza, and rice (*Lean Cuisine*), 9 oz. 290
Enchilada sauce:
(*Chi-Chi's*), ¼ cup 30
(*La Victoria*), ¼ cup 20
Enchilada seasoning mix (*Lawry's*), 2 tsp. 20
Endive, chopped, ½ cup 4
Eppaw, ½ cup 75
Escarole, see "Endive"
Etouffée dinner mix (*Luzianne*), ¼ pkg. 200

F

FOOD AND MEASURE	CALORIES
Fajita entree, frozen:	
beef (*Tyson* Kit), 3.6-oz. fajita	130
chicken (*Healthy Choice* Fiesta), 7 oz.	260
chicken (*Tyson* Kit), 3.6-oz. fajita	120
Fajita sauce, 2 tbsp., except as noted:	
cooking (*S&W* Southwestern), 1 tbsp.	10
and marinade (*World Harbors* Guadalupe)	45
skillet (*Lawry's*), 2 tbsp.	15
Fajita seasoning mix:	
(*Lawry's*), 2 tsp.	15
beef (*Durkee* Easy), 1/6 pkg.	15
Falafel mix:	
(*Fantastic Falafil*), 1/2 cup	250
(*Near East*), 2 1/2 fried patties*	230
Farina, whole grain, cooked (see also "Cereal"), 1 cup	116
Farina, whole grain, dry, 1 oz.	105
Fava beans, see "Broad beans"	
Feijoa, raw (*Frieda's*), 1 oz.	17
Fennel, bulb, raw, trimmed, sliced, 1/2 cup	27
Fettuccine, plain, dry, see "Pasta"	
Fettuccine, refrigerated (*Contadina*), 1 1/4 cup	250
Fettuccine entree, frozen:	
Alfredo (*Banquet*), 10.5 oz.	370
Alfredo (*Healthy Choice*), 8 oz.	250
Alfredo (*Lean Cuisine*), 9 oz.	270
Alfredo (*Marie Callender's*), 1 cup	350
Alfredo (*Stouffer's*), 10 oz.	580
Alfredo, with broccoli (*Weight Watchers*), 8.5 oz.	230
with broccoli and chicken (*Marie Callender's*), 1 cup	420
chicken, see "Chicken entree"	
primavera (*Lean Cuisine*), 10 oz.	260
primavera (*Marie Callender's*), 1 cup	310
primavera (*Stouffer's Lunch Express*), 10 1/4 oz.	420

Fettuccine entree mix:
(*Noodle Roni*), 1 cup* 470
with creamy basil sauce (*Knorr* Cup), 1 pkg. 220
Fig:
fresh, 1 medium, 1.8 oz. 37
canned, whole, Kadota (*S&W*), 5 pieces 140
dried, Calamata string (*Agora*), ½ cup 250
dried, California, 4 figs, 2 oz. 143
dried, Calimyrna or Mission (*Blue Ribbon/Sun·Maid*),
4 figs, 1.5 oz. 120
dried, white or mission (*Sonoma*), 3–4 figs, 1.4 oz. . . . 110
Filberts, salted or unsalted:
dried, 1 oz. 179
dry-roasted or oil-roasted, 1 oz. 188
Fillo pastry, frozen (*Apollo*), ⅛ pkg. 180
Fish, see specific listings
Fish dinner, frozen (see also specific fish listings):
battered portions, 'n chips (*Swanson*), 1 pkg. 480
breaded sticks (*Swanson* Budget), 1 pkg. 340
Fish entree, frozen (see also specific fish listings):
(*Van de Kamp's* Fish 'n Fries), 6.5 oz. 380
baked, with shells (*Lean Cuisine*), 9 oz. 260
cakes (*Mrs. Paul's*), 2 pieces 200
and chips (*Swanson*), 1 pkg. 310
fillets, battered (*Mrs. Paul's* Crunchy), 2 pieces 250
fillets, breaded (*Mrs. Paul's*), 2 pieces 240
fillets, in lemon pepper sauce (*Healthy Choice*), 10.7 oz. 290
grilled, with vegetables (*Lean Cuisine* Cafe Classics),
8⅞ oz. 170
with macaroni and cheese (*Swanson*), 1 pkg. 350
portions, battered (*Mrs. Paul's*), 2 pieces 280
portions, breaded (*Mrs. Paul's*), 2 pieces 190
sticks, battered (*Mrs. Paul's*), 6 pieces 240
sticks, breaded (*Mrs. Paul's*), 6 pieces 220
sticks, breaded, crisp (*Mrs. Paul's* Crispy Crunchy),
5 pieces 200
Fish sandwich, fillet, with cheese, frozen (*Mrs. Paul's*),
1 piece 330

Fish seasoning and coating mix (*Shake 'n Bake*), 1/4 pkt. 7
Flatbread, see "Cracker"
Flatfish, meat only, baked, broiled, or microwaved, 4 oz. 133
Flax seeds (*Arrowhead Mills*), 3 tbsp., 1 oz. 140
Flounder, fresh, see "Flatfish"
Flounder entree, fillets, frozen:
battered (*Mrs. Paul's* Crunchy), 2 pieces 260
breaded (*Mrs. Paul's* Premium), 1 piece 240
Flour, see "Wheat flour" and specific flour listings
Frankfurter, (see also "Chicken frankfurter" and "Turkey frankfurter"):
(*Hormel* 10), 1.6-oz. link 140
(*Hormel* 8/*Hormel* Big 8), 2-oz. link 180
(*Oscar Mayer* Wieners), 1.6-oz. link 150
all varieties (*Wranglers*), 2-oz. link 170
beef:
(*Boar's Head* Giant), 2 oz. 160
(*Boar's Head* Skinless), 1.6 oz. 120
(*Hebrew National*), 1.7 oz. 150
(*Hebrew National* Family Pack), 2 oz. 180
(*Hebrew National* 8 oz.), 1.7 oz. 140
(*Hebrew National* Reduced Fat), 1.7 oz. 120
(*Hormel* 8), 2 oz. 170
(*Oscar Mayer* Light), 2 oz. 110
(*Oscar Mayer Big & Juicy* Original), 2.7 oz. 240
(*Oscar Mayer Bun-Length*), 2 oz. 190
beef or cheese (*Oscar Mayer*), 1.6-oz. link 140
cocktail (*Hormel* Wieners), 5 links 160
cocktail, smoked (*Hormel* Smokies), 5 links 180
hot and spicy or smoked (*Oscar Mayer Big & Juicy*), 2.7-oz. link 220
light, regular or beef (*Hormel Light & Lean 97*), 1.6-oz. link 45
"Frankfurter," vegetarian, 1 link:
frozen (*Morningstar Farms* Deli Franks) 110
frozen (*Natural Touch* Vege) 100
frozen (*Worthington Leanies*) 110
frozen, corn battered (*Loma Linda* Corn Dog) 220

"Frankfurter," vegetarian *(cont.)*
refrigerated, chili (*Yves Veggie Cuisine* Dogs) 70
refrigerated, tofu (*Yves Veggie Cuisine* Weiners) 57
Frankfurter sandwich, frozen, 1 piece, except as noted:
(*Hormel Quick Meal* Jumbo Dog) 350
bagel wrapped (*Boar's Head* Bagel Dog) 310
bagel wrapped (*Hebrew National* Bagel Dog) 400
with cheese (*Hormel Quick Meal* Cheesey Dog) 310
chili, with cheese (*Hormel Quick Meal*) 350
corn dog (*Hormel/Hormel Quick Meal*) 220
corn dog, mini (*Hormel Quick Meal*), 5 pieces 250
French toast, frozen:
(*Downyflake*), 2 pieces 260
regular or cinnamon (*Aunt Jemima*), 2 pieces 240
French toast breakfast, frozen, 1 pkg.:
cinnamon swirl (*Swanson Great Starts*) 440
with sausage (*Swanson Great Starts*) 410
Frosting, ready-to-spread, 2 tbsp.:
caramel pecan (*Pillsbury Supreme/Creamy Supreme*) . . . 150
chocolate or milk chocolate (*Betty Crocker Creamy Deluxe*) 150
chocolate, all flavors except dark (*Pillsbury Supreme/Creamy Supreme*) 140
chocolate, dark (*Pillsbury Supreme/Creamy Supreme*) . . 130
chocolate, Swiss almond (*Betty Crocker Creamy Deluxe*) 150
coconut, almond or pecan (*Pillsbury Supreme*) 160
cookie (*Pillsbury Supreme/Creamy Supreme Oreo*) 150
cream cheese (*Betty Crocker Creamy Deluxe*) 140
lemon or strawberry creme (*Pillsbury Supreme/Creamy Supreme*) 150
rainbow chip (*Betty Crocker Creamy Deluxe*) 160
vanilla or French vanilla (*Betty Crocker Creamy Deluxe*) 140
Frozen desserts, see "Ice cream" and "Ice cream desserts"
Fruit, see specific listings
Fruit, mixed, candied (*S&W* Glace), 2 tbsp. 90
Fruit, mixed, canned (see also "Fruit cocktail"), ½ cup:
in juice, chunky (*Libby's* Lite) 60
in heavy syrup, chunky (*Del Monte*) 100

tropical salad, in light syrup (*Dole*) 80
Fruit, mixed, dried (*Dole Sun Giant*), 1.5 oz. 100
Fruit bar, frozen (see also "Yogurt bar, frozen"):
all flavors (*Dole*), 1.75-oz. bar .45
all flavors (*Dole* No Sugar), 1.75-oz. bar 25
all flavors except coconut (*Edy's*), 1 bar 90
all flavors (*Starburst*), 1 bar 50
coconut (*Edy's* Calypso), 1 bar 190
Fruit cocktail, canned, ½ cup:
(*Del Monte* Very Cherry) 90
(*Hunt's*) 90
in juice (*Libby's* Lite) 60
in heavy syrup (*S&W*) 90
Fruit dip, chocolate or caramel (*Smucker's* Fat Free),
2 tbsp. 130
Fruit drink blends (see also specific listings):
(*Dole* Fruit Fiesta), 16 fl. oz. 270
(*Dole* Lanai/Tropical Breeze), 16 fl. oz. 240
(*Snapple* Bali Blast/Samoan Splash), 8 fl. oz. 120
frozen* (*Dole* Fruit Fiesta), 8 fl. oz. 140
frozen* (*Dole* Lanai/Tropical Breeze), 8 fl. oz. 120
nectar (*Kern's* Tropical), 11.5 fl. oz. 210
punch (*Dole* Paradise), 10 fl. oz. 150
punch (*Dole* Tropical), 10 fl. oz. 130
punch (*Snapple*), 8 fl. oz. 110
punch, frozen* (*Minute Maid*), 8 fl. oz. 120
Fruit juice blends (see also specific fruit listings):
(*R.W. Knudsen* Morning Blend/Vita), 8 fl. oz. 120
(*R.W. Knudsen* Natural Breakfast), 8 fl. oz. 110
(*Snapple* Vitamin Supreme), 10 fl. oz. 150
punch or tropical (*Juicy Juice*), 8 fl. oz. 130
tropical fruit (*Juicy Juice*), 8 fl. oz. 130
Fruit and nut mix, see "Trail mix"
Fruit roll or snack, all varieties (*Fruit Roll Ups*), 1 oz. . . 110
Fruit spreads (see also "Jam and preserves"):
all varieties (*Kraft* Reduced Calorie), 1 tbsp. 20
all varieties (*Polaner*), 1 tbsp. 40
all varieties (*R.W. Knudsen*), 1 tbsp. 50

Fruit syrup (see also specific fruit listings):
(*Smucker's* Natural), 1/4 cup 210
light (*Smucker's*), 1/4 cup 130
and maple (*R.W. Knudsen*), 1/4 cup 150
Fusilli pasta mix, with creamy pesto (*Knorr*), 2/3 cup . . . 250

G

FOOD AND MEASURE	CALORIES
Garbanzo beans, see "Chickpeas"	
Garden salad, canned, dill or marinated (*S&W*), ½ cup	50
Garlic:	
1 clove, approx. .1 oz.	4
crushed (*Christopher Ranch*), 1 tsp.	10
Garlic, pickled (*Christopher Ranch*), 3 pieces, ¼ oz.	5
Garlic dip, 2 tbsp.:	
(*Nalley's*)	130
creamy Italian (*Marie's*), 2 tbsp.	180
roasted, and onion (*Marie's* Fat Free), 2 tbsp.	35
Garlic dressing (*Christopher Ranch*), 1 tbsp.	53
Garlic pickle, relish (*Patak's*), 1 tbsp.	45
Garlic powder (*Tone's*), ¼ tsp.	5
Garlic salt (*Lawry's*), ¼ tsp.	0
Garlic spread:	
(*Lawry's* Concentrate), 2 tsp.	50
(*Lawry's* Ready-to-Spread), 1 tbsp.	100
Garlic sprouts (*Jonathan's*), 1 cup, 4 oz.	70
Garlic and basil, chopped (*Paesana*), 1 tsp.	6
Gefilte fish, drained:	
(*Manischewitz* Gold/Jelled Broth), 1 ball, with jell	110
zesty (*Manischewitz* Gold/Brine), 1 ball	70
Gelatin, unflavored (*Knox*), 1 pkt.	25
Gelatin dessert, 3.5 oz.:	
all flavors (*Del Monte* Snack)	70
all flavors (*Hunt's Snack Pack*)	100
all flavors (*Jell-O* Snacks)	80
Gelatin dessert mix*, ½ cup:	
all flavors (*Jell-O*), ½ cup	80
all flavors (*Jell-O* Sugar Free), ½ cup	10
strawberry (*Jell-O 1-2-3*), ⅔ cup	130
Giardiniera, see "Vegetables, mixed, pickled"	
Ginger, fresh, trimmed root, sliced, ¼ cup	17

Ginger, candied or crystallized (*Paradise/White Swan*), 1 oz. 100
Ginger, pickled, Japanese, 1 oz. 10
Ginger juice drink (*Santa Cruz* Hawaiian), 8 fl. oz. 110
Ginkgo nut, shelled, canned, drained, 1 oz. 32
Glaze, fruit:
for banana, creamy (*Marie's*), 2 tbsp. 60
for blueberries, peaches, or strawberries (*Marie's*), 2 tbsp. 40
for pie, strawberry (*Smucker's*), 2 oz. 80
Glaze, ham, see "Ham glaze"
Goat, meat only, roasted, 4 oz. 162
Godfather's Pizza, 1 slice:
cheese, original crust:
mini, 1/4 pie 138
small, 1/6 pie 239
medium, 1/8 pie 242
large, 1/10 pie 271
cheese, golden crust:
small, 1/6 pie 213
medium, 1/8 pie 229
large, 1/10 pie 261
combo, original crust:
mini, 1/4 pie 164
small, 1/6 pie 299
medium, 1/8 pie 318
large, 1/10 pie 332
combo, golden crust:
small, 1/6 pie 273
medium, 1/8 pie 283
large, 1/10 pie 322
Goose, domesticated:
roasted, meat with skin, 4 oz. 346
roasted, meat only, 4 oz. 270
Goose liver, see "Pâté"
Gooseberry:
fresh, 1/2 cup 34
fresh, green (*Frieda's*), 1 oz. 11
canned, in light syrup, 1/2 cup 93

Gorgonzola sauce, refrigerated (*Monterey Pasta Company*), 4 oz. 400
Goulash seasoning mix (*Knorr* Recipe), 1⅓ tbsp. 35
Grains, see specific listings
Granola, see "Cereal"
Granola and cereal bar 1 bar:
all varieties (*Health Valley* Fat Free Granola Bar) 140
all varieties (*Health Valley Healthy Energy Bars*) 180
blueberry (*Kudos* Low Fat) 90
chocolate chip (*Carnation* Chewy) 150
chocolate chip (*Kudos* Enrobed) 120
chocolate chip (*Kudos* Unenrobed) 90
fudge, nutty (*Kudos*) 130
milk and cookies (*Kudos*) 130
oats and honey (*Carnation* Granola) 130
peanut butter (*Kudos*) 130
peanut butter–chocolate chip (*Carnation* Chewy) 150
strawberry (*Kudos* Low Fat) 80
Grape:
fresh, American type (slipskin) 10 medium 15
fresh, European type (adherent skin) seedless, 10 medium 36
canned, Thompson seedless, in heavy syrup (*S&W*), ½ cup 100
Grape drink:
(*Capri Sun*), 6.75 fl. oz. 110
(*Dole*), 10 fl. oz. 150
(*Snapple* Grapeade), 8 fl. oz. 110
(*Veryfine* Glacial), 8 fl. oz. 110
frozen* (*Minute Maid* Drink/Punch), 8 fl. oz. 120
Grape drink blend:
apple (*Tree Top*), 11.5 fl. oz. 190
punch (*Minute Maid*), 8 fl. oz. 120
Grape juice, 8 fl. oz.:
(*After the Fall* Concord) 130
(*Juicy Juice*) 130
(*Lucky Leaf*) 140
(*R.W. Knudsen*) 150
(*R.W. Knudsen* Concord) 160

Grape juice ***(cont.)***
(*Veryfine*) 180
(*Veryfine* Juice-Ups) 130
Grape leaves, in jars:
(*Krinos*), 1 leaf 5
stuffed, with rice (*Perfecta* Dolmadakia Yalandji), 4.35 oz. 220
Grapefruit:
fresh, pink or red, California or Arizona, ½ medium, 3¾″ diam. 46
fresh, pink or red, Florida, ½ medium, 3¾″ diam. 37
fresh, white, California, ½ medium, 3¾″ diam. 43
fresh, white, Florida, ½ medium or ½-cup sections with juice 38
canned or (*S&W* Natural Style), ⅔ cup 50
Grapefruit drink, pink, 8 fl. oz.
(*Tree Top* Desert Ice) 120
(*Tropicana Twister*) 120
Grapefruit juice, 8 fl. oz., except as noted:
(*Dole*), 10 fl. oz. 120
(*Tree Top*) 100
(*Veryfine*) 90
blend (*Dole* Sunripe) 130
blend, cranberry (*Apple & Eve* Ruby Red) 120
frozen* (*Minute Maid*), 8 fl. oz. 100
golden (*Tropicana*) 90
pink or white (*R.W. Knudsen*) 100
red (*R.W. Knudsen* Rio) 140
Gravy, see specific listings
Great northern beans, ½ cup:
dry, boiled 104
canned (*Allens*) 100
canned (*Stokely*) 110
canned, with sausage (*Trappey's*) 100
Green beans, ½ cup, except as noted:
fresh, raw 17
fresh, boiled, drained 22
canned (*Stokely/Stokely* No Salt) 20
canned, whole, cut, or French (*S&W*) 20
canned, dilled (*S&W*), 1 oz. 20

canned, and wax beans (*S&W*) 20
frozen (*Seabrook*), 1 cup 25
Greens, mixed, canned (*Allens/Sunshine*), ½ cup 30
Grenadine syrup (*Rose's*), 1 tbsp. 32
Grilling sauce (see also specific listings):
chardonnay or Tuscan herb (*Knorr*), 2 tbsp. 35
mandarin ginger (*Knorr* Microwave), 2 tbsp. 45
Parmesano (*Knorr* Microwave), 3 tbsp. 50
plum, spicy (*Knorr*), 2 tbsp. 50
tequila lime (*Knorr*), 2 tbsp. 40
Grits, see "Corn grits"
Ground cherry, trimmed, ½ cup 37
Grouper, meat only, baked, broiled, or microwaved, 4 oz. 134
Guacamole dip, spicy (*Nalley's*), 2 tbsp. 120
Guacamole seasoning (*Lawry's*), ½ tsp. 5
Guanabana, frozen, chunks (*Goya*), ⅓ pkg. 60
Guanabana nectar, canned (*Goya*), 12 fl. oz. 230
Guava:
fresh, ½ cup 42
fresh, strawberry, ½ cup 85
Guava drink (*Snapple* Guava Mania), 8 fl. oz. 110
Guava juice (*After the Fall* Guava Maya), 8 fl. oz. 110
Guava nectar:
(*Kern's*), 8 fl. oz. 150
(*Libby's/Kern's*), 11.5 fl. oz. 220
Guava paste (*Goya*), ¾" slice 100
Gumbo dinner mix (*Luzianne*), ⅕ pkg. 160
Gyro mix (*Casbah*), ⅒ pkg. 64

H

FOOD AND MEASURE	CALORIES
Häagen-Dazs Ice Cream Shop, ½ cup:	
ice cream:	
cappuccino	270
cherry, brandied	250
chocolate, Belgian	330
chocolate Swiss almond or coffee chip	300
macadamia nut or maple walnut	330
pralines and cream	290
vanilla chip	300
sorbet, lemon or orange	140
sorbet, raspberry	110
yogurt, soft serve:	
chocolate	120
coffee or raspberry	140
strawberry	120
vanilla	110
Haddock, baked, broiled, or microwaved, 4 oz.	127
Haddock, smoked, 4 oz.	132
Haddock entree, frozen:	
battered (*Mrs. Paul's* Crunchy), 2 pieces	250
breaded (*Mrs. Paul's* Premium), 1 piece	230
Halibut, meat only, 4 oz.:	
fresh, Atlantic and Pacific, baked, broiled, or microwaved	159
fresh, Greenland, baked, broiled, or microwaved	271
frozen, fillet or steaks (*Peter Pan*)	110
Halibut entree, frozen, battered (*Van de Kamp's*), 3 pieces	300
Ham, meat only, 4 oz.:	
fresh, whole leg, lean with fat, roasted	333
fresh, whole leg, lean only, roasted	249
cured, whole leg, lean with fat, roasted	276
cured, whole leg, lean only, roasted	178
cured, boneless (11% fat), roasted	202

cured, boneless, extra lean (5% fat), roasted 164
Ham, canned or refrigerated, 3 oz.:
(*Hormel Light & Lean*) 90
(*John Morrell* Boneless) 140
Black Forest (*Boar's Head* Baby) 90
maple (*Boar's Head Baby Honey Coat*) 90
slice, smoked or maple glaze (*Boar's Head Sweet Slice*) 110
smoked, semi-boneless (*Boar's Head*) 130
spiral sliced (*Spiral Cure 81* Half) 150
steak, honey (*Patrick Cudahy*) 100
steak, smoke flavor (*Patrick Cudahy*) 90
Virginia (*Boar's Head* Ready-to-Eat) 100
Virginia, smoked (*Boar's Head* Baby Gourmet) 90
Ham bologna (*Boar's Head*), 2 oz. 80
Ham glaze (*Crosse & Blackwell*), 1 tbsp. 30
Ham lunch meat:
(*Boar's Head* Deluxe), 2 oz. 60
(*Jones Dairy Farm Lean Choice*), 2 slices 50
all varieties except apple (*Healthy Deli*), 2 oz. 60
all varieties (*Hormel Light & Lean* 97 Deli), 2 oz. 50
apple (*Healthy Deli* Cinnamon Apple Grove), 2 oz. 70
baked (*Louis Rich Carving Board*), 2 slices, 1.8 oz. 50
baked, boiled, or smoked (*Oscar Mayer*), 3 slices, 2.2 oz. . 60
baked, Virginia (*Healthy Deli* Less Sodium), 2 oz. 70
Black Forest (*Boar's Head*), 2 oz. 60
cappicola (*Boar's Head* Cappy), 2 oz. 60
chopped (*Black Label*), 2 oz. 140
maple (*Boar's Head Honey Coat*), 2 oz. 60
pepper (*Boar's Head*), 2 oz. 70
smoked (*Boar's Head* Gourmet), 2 oz. 60
smoked (*Louis Rich Carving Board*), 2 slices, 1.6 oz. 45
spiced (*Boar's Head*), 2 oz. 120
Virginia (*Healthy Deli*), 2 oz. 60
Ham patty (*Hormel*), 2-oz. patty 180
Ham spread:
(*Libby's Spreadables*), 1/3 cup 110
deviled (*Cure 81*), 2 oz. 150
deviled (*Underwood*), 1/4 cup 160
Ham and cheese loaf (*Oscar Mayer*), 1 oz. 70

Ham and cheese patty (*Hormel*), 2-oz. patty 190
Ham and cheese sandwich, frozen, 1 piece:
(*Croissant Pockets*) 360
(*Hormel Quick Meal*) 330
(*Hot Pockets*) 340
Hamburger, see "Beef sandwich"
"Hamburger," vegetarian, frozen, 1 patty:
(*Amy's* California), 2.5 oz. 100
(*Amy's* Chicago), 2.5 oz. 160
(*Green Giant Harvest Burgers* Original) 140
(*Ken & Robert's Veggie Burger*), 2.5 oz. 130
Italian or southwestern (*Green Giant Harvest Burgers*) . . 140
Hamburger entree mix, dry:
beef pasta (*Hamburger Helper*), 2/3 cup 120
beef taco or zesty Italian (*Hamburger Helper*), 1/2 cup . . . 160
cheeseburger macaroni (*Hamburger Helper*), 1/3 cup . . . 180
chili or with cheese (*Hamburger Mate*), 1/5 pkg. 160
fettuccine Alfredo (*Hamburger Helper*), 1/2 cup 140
lasagna (*Hamburger Helper*), 2/3 cup 140
with noodles (*Hamburger Mate*), 1/5 pkg. 150
pizza pasta (*Hamburger Helper*), 1/2 cup 150
Stroganoff (*Hamburger Helper*), 2/3 cup 170
Hardee's, 1 serving:
breakfast items:
Big Country Breakfast, bacon 820
Big Country Breakfast, sausage 1000
biscuit, apple cinnamon and raisin 200
biscuit, bacon and egg 530
biscuit, bacon, egg, and cheese 610
biscuit, country ham 430
biscuit, ham 400
biscuit, ham, egg, and cheese 540
biscuit, *Rise 'N' Shine* 190
biscuit, sausage 510
biscuit, sausage and egg 600
Biscuit 'N' Gravy 510
Frisco Breakfast Sandwich, ham 500
hash rounds, regular 230
pancakes, 3 cakes 280

ultimate omelet 530
burgers:
bacon cheeseburger 530
cheeseburger 390
cheeseburger, ¼ lb. 420
cheeseburger, big double 630
Big Hardee 590
Big Hardee, with cheese 690
Frisco burger 740
hamburger 340
Hardee Jr. 400
Hardee Jr., with cheese 450
Mushroom 'N' Swiss 610
sandwiches:
chicken, grilled 290
chicken fillet 420
Fisherman's Fillet 450
Hot Ham 'N' Cheese 300
roast beef, big 410
roast beef, regular 270
chicken:
breast 370
leg 170
thigh 330
wing 200
salads:
garden 220
grilled chicken 150
side salad 25
dressings:
French, fat free 70
ranch 290
Thousand Island 250
side dishes:
baked beans, 5 oz. 170
coleslaw, 4 oz. 240
fries, small 240
fries, medium 350
fries, large 430

Hardee's*, side dishes *(cont.)
gravy, 1.5 oz. 20
mashed potato, 4 oz. 70
desserts and shakes:
Big Cookie 280
Cool Twist cone, chocolate 180
Cool Twist cone, vanilla 170
Cool Twist cone, vanilla/chocolate 180
Cool Twist sundae, hot fudge 290
Cool Twist sundae, strawberry 210
peach cobbler, 6 oz. 310
shake, chocolate 370
shake, peach 390
shake, strawberry 420
shake, vanilla 350
Hash (see also specific listings), canned (*Mary Kitchen* Fiesta), 1 cup 210
Hazelnut, see "Filberts"
Hazelnut butter (*Roaster Fresh*), 1 oz. 188
Head cheese (*Oscar Mayer*), 1-oz. slice 50
Herring, fresh, 4 oz.:
Atlantic, meat only, baked, broiled, or microwaved 230
Atlantic, meat only, kippered 246
Atlantic, meat only, pickled 297
Pacific, meat only, baked, broiled, or microwaved 284
Herring, in jars, drained:
(*Vita* Homestyle) 2 oz. 130
in sour cream (*Vita*), 1/4 cup, 2 1/4 oz. 120
roll mops (*Vita*), 2 1/2 oz., about 1 piece 140
Herring salad (*Vita*), 1/4 cup 110
Hickory nut, dried, shelled, 1 oz. 187
Hoisin sauce (*Lee Kum Kee*), 2 tbsp. 100
Hollandaise sauce mix (*Knorr*), 1/10 pkg., 1 tsp. 10
Homestyle gravy mix (*French's*), 1/4 cup* 10
Hominy (see also "Corn grits"), canned:
golden (*Goya*), 1/2 cup 120
golden (*Sun-Vista*), 1/2 cup 70
Mexican (*Allens/Uncle William*), 1/2 cup 120
white (*Goya*), 1/2 cup 100

white (*Sun-Vista*) 1/2 cup 65
Honey (*Aunt Sue's/Grandma's/Sue Bee*), 1 tbsp. 60
Honey butter (*Downey's*), .5 oz. 60
Honey mustard sauce, California style (*Rice Road*),
1 tbsp. 20
Honeydew:
fresh, 1/10 melon, 7″ × 2″ 46
fresh, pulp, cubed, 1/2 cup 30
Horseradish, prepared:
(*Heluva* Good), 1 tsp. 0
red (*Rosoff*), 1 tbsp. 8
white (*Rosoff*), 1 tbsp. 7
Horseradish sauce (*Heinz*), 1 tsp. 25
Hot dog, see "Frankfurter"
Hubbard squash:
fresh, baked, cubed, 1/2 cup 51
fresh, boiled, drained, mashed, 1/2 cup 35
Hummus (*Casbah*), 1 oz. 85
Hummus dip mix (*Fantastic Foods*), 2 tbsp.* 60

I

FOOD AND MEASURE	CALORIES
Ice, Italian (see also "Sorbet"), 6 fl. oz.:	
all flavors, except cherry and chocolate fudge (*Luigi's*)	110
cherry (*Luigi's*)	120
chocolate fudge (*Luigi's*)	150
Ice cream, ½ cup:	
almond praline or butter pecan (*Edy's Grand*)	160
amaretto (*Häagen-Dazs DiSaronno*)	260
banana split or chocolate fudge sundae (*Edy's Grand*)	170
(*Ben & Jerry's Chubby Hubby*)	350
(*Ben & Jerry's Chunky Monkey*)	280
(*Ben & Jerry's Rainforest Crunch*)	300
(*Ben & Jerry's Wavy Gravy*)	330
brownie, double fudge (*Edy's Grand*)	160
brownie batter or cherry chocolate chip (*Edy's Grand*)	150
Brownies à la Mode (*Häagen-Dazs Extrāas*)	280
butter pecan (*Ben & Jerry's*)	310
butter pecan (*Häagen-Dazs*)	320
Caramel Cone Explosion (*Häagen-Dazs Extrāas*)	310
cherry chocolate chip (*Ben & Jerry's Cherry Garcia*)	240
chocolate or coffee (*Edy's Grand*)	140
chocolate, vanilla, or coffee (*Häagen-Dazs*)	270
chocolate chip, regular or mint (*Edy's Grand* Chips!)	160
chocolate chip cookie dough (*Ben & Jerry's*)	270
chocolate chocolate chip (*Edy's Grand*)	160
chocolate chocolate chip (*Häagen-Dazs*)	300
chocolate cookie, mint (*Ben & Jerry's*)	260
coffee (*Ben & Jerry's Cafe Olé*)	230
coffee fudge, almond (*Ben & Jerry's*)	290
cookies and cream (*Häagen-Dazs*)	270
cookies and cream or ice cream sandwich (*Edy's Grand*)	150
cookie dough or rocky road (*Edy's Grand*)	170
Cookie Dough Dynamo (*Häagen-Dazs Extrāas*)	300
espresso chip (*Edy's Grand*)	150

fudge chunk (*Ben & Jerry's* New York Super) 290
Irish cream (*Häagen-Dazs Baileys*) 280
macadamia brittle (*Häagen-Dazs*) 300
mocha fudge (*Ben & Jerry's*) 270
Peanut Butter Burst (*Häagen-Dazs Exträas*) 330
peanut butter cup (*Ben & Jerry's*) 370
rum raisin (*Häagen-Dazs*) 270
strawberry (*Edy's Grand*) 130
strawberry (*Häagen-Dazs*) 250
strawberry cheesecake chunk (*Edy's Grand*) 150
Strawberry Cheesecake Craze (*Häagen-Dazs Exträas*) . . . 290
toffee crunch, coffee or English (*Ben & Jerry's*) 280
Triple Brownie Overload (*Häagen-Dazs Exträas*) 300
vanilla (*Ben & Jerry's*) 230
vanilla or vanilla bean (*Edy's Grand*) 150
vanilla, French (*Edy's Grand*) 160
vanilla caramel, fudge swirl (*Ben & Jerry's*) 280
vanilla, chocolate, strawberry (*Edy's Grand*) 130
vanilla fudge (*Häagen-Dazs*) 280
vanilla Swiss almond (*Häagen-Dazs*) 310

"Ice cream," imitation, (see also " 'Ice cream,' tofu"):
bar, chocolate (*Rice Dream*), 1 bar 270
bar, nutty, chocolate or vanilla (*Rice Dream*), 1 bar 260
bar, strawberry (*Rice Dream*), 1 bar 250
cappuccino or lemon (*Rice Dream*), ½ cup 130
carob, carob chip, or mint carob chip (*Rice Dream*),
½ cup 130
carob, almond (*Rice Dream*), ½ cup 140
cocoa marble fudge or peanut butter fudge (*Rice Dream*), ½ cup 130
cookies n' dream (*Rice Dream*), ½ cup 140
Neapolitan (*Rice Dream*), ½ cup 120
strawberry or wildberry (*Rice Dream*), ½ cup 110
vanilla, vanilla fudge, or vanilla Swiss almond (*Rice Dream*), ½ cup 130

"Ice cream," tofu:
all fruit flavors (*Tofutti Fruit*), ½ cup 100
better pecan (*Tofutti*), ½ cup 220
chocolate (*Tofutti*), ½ cup 180

"Ice cream," tofu *(cont.)*
chocolate cake (*Tofutti*), ½ cup 210
sandwich, chocolate (*Tofutti Cuties*), 1 piece 130
sandwich, vanilla or wildberry (*Tofutti Cuties*), 1 piece . . 121
soft serve, all flavors (*Tofutti*), ½ cup 190
soft serve, light, all flavors (*Tofutti* Lite), ½ cup 90
stick, chocolate (*Tofutti Frutti*), 1 bar 120
stick, fudge (*Tofutti* Teddy), 1 bar 70
vanilla or vanilla fudge (*Tofutti*), ½ cup 190
vanilla, almond bark (*Tofutti*), ½ cup 210
wildberry (*Tofutti*), ½ cup 190

Ice cream bar, 1 bar:
almond (*DoveBar*) 280
almond (*DoveBar* Single) 350
(*Butterfinger*) 190
Caramel Cone Explosion (*Häagen-Dazs Exträas*) 350
caramel creme with toffee chips (*DoveBar*) 280
chocolate or vanilla (*Nestlé Crunch*) 200
chocolate (*3 Musketeers*) 140
chocolate, dark (*Häagen-Dazs*) 400
chocolate cookie dough (*Ben & Jerry's*) 420
Cookie Dough Dynamo (*Häagen-Dazs Exträas*) 380
coffee with almond crunch (*Häagen-Dazs*) 360
Iced Cappuccino (*Häagen-Dazs Exträas*) 330
(*Klondike* Original) 290
(*Milky Way*) 140
mocha cashew crunch (*DoveBar*) 260
peppermint with dark chocolate (*DoveBar*) 290
(*Snickers*) 190
toffee crunch, English (*Ben & Jerry's*) 330
Triple Brownie Overload (*Häagen-Dazs Exträas*) 380
vanilla (*Ben & Jerry's*) 330
vanilla (*3 Musketeers*) 190
vanilla, almond (*Häagen-Dazs*) 370
vanilla, brownie (*Ben & Jerry's*) 330
vanilla, dark or milk chocolate coated (*DoveBar*) 260
vanilla, dark chocolate-coated (*Häagen-Dazs*) 400
vanilla, milk chocolate-coated (*Häagen-Dazs*) 330
vanilla, white coated (*DoveBar*) 270

Ice cream cone, filled, 1 cone:
chocolate or chocolate dipped (*Drumstick*) 320
vanilla (*Drumstick*) 340
vanilla caramel or fudge (*Drumstick*) 360
Ice cream cup, filled:
chocolate (*Carnation*), 3 fl. oz. 140
chocolate malt (*Carnation*), 12 fl. oz. 270
chocolate sundae (*Carnation*), 5 fl. oz. 210
strawberry or vanilla (*Carnation*), 3 fl. oz. 100
strawberry sundae (*Carnation*), 5 fl. oz. 200
Ice cream desserts:
chocolate malt (*Milky Way*), 1 cup 220
loaf, all flavors (*Viennetta*), 1/5 of 12-oz. pkg. 190
nuggets, chocolate coated (*Nestlé Crunch*), 8 pieces . . . 310
Ice cream sandwich, 1 piece:
chocolate chip cookie (*Chipwich* Jr.) 240
(*Klondike* Big Bear) 200
(*Klondike* Krispy) 300
Italian beans, in sauce, canned (*Green Giant/Joan of Arc*), 1/2 cup 130

J

FOOD AND MEASURE	CALORIES
Jack-in-the-Box, 1 serving:	
breakfast:	
Breakfast Jack	300
Country Crock Spread, .2 oz.	25
croissant, sausage	670
croissant, supreme	570
hash browns	160
pancake platter	400
pancake syrup, 1.5 oz.	120
sandwich, breakfast, sourdough	380
sandwich, breakfast, ultimate	620
scrambled egg pocket	430
sandwiches and burgers:	
beef, Monterey roast	540
cheeseburger, regular	320
cheeseburger, double	450
cheeseburger, ultimate	1030
cheeseburger, bacon bacon	710
cheeseburger, Colossus	1100
cheeseburger, *The Outlaw Burger*	720
chicken	400
chicken, Caesar	520
chicken, spicy crispy	560
chicken, supreme	620
chicken fajita pita	290
chicken fillet, grilled	430
The Really Big Chicken Sandwich	900
fish supreme	590
hamburger, regular	280
hamburger, quarter pounder	510
hamburger, sourdough, grilled	670
Jumbo Jack	560
Jumbo Jack with cheese	650

chicken teriyaki bowl 580
taco 190
taco, super 280
salad, chicken, garden 200
salad, side 70
finger foods:
  chicken strips, 4 pieces 290
  chicken strips, 6 pieces 450
  egg rolls, 3 pieces 440
  egg rolls, 5 pieces 750
  jalapeños, stuffed, 7 pieces 420
  jalapeños, stuffed, 10 pieces 600
  potato wedges, with bacon and cheddar 800
side dishes:
  fries, small 220
  fries, regular 350
  fries, jumbo 400
  fries, super scoop 590
  fries, seasoned, curly 360
  onion rings 380
sauces and dressings:
  barbecue sauce, 1 oz. 45
  blue cheese dressing, 2 oz. 210
  buttermilk dressing, house, 2 oz. 290
  buttermilk sauce, .9 oz. 130
  Italian dressing, low calorie, 2 oz. 25
  sweet and sour sauce, 1 oz. 40
  tartar sauce, 1 oz. 150
  Thousand Island dressing, 2 oz. 250
desserts and shakes:
  apple turnover 350
  cheesecake 310
  cheesecake, chocolate chip cookie dough 360
  shake, chocolate 390
  shake, strawberry 330
  shake, vanilla 350
Jackfruit, trimmed, 1 oz. .27
Jalapeño, see "Pepper, jalapeño"
Jalapeño dip, see "Bean dip" and "Cheese dip"

Jam and preserves (see also "Fruit spreads"), 1 tbsp.:
all varieties (*Smucker's*) 50
all varieties (*Smucker's* Reduced Sugar) 25
all varieties (*Smucker's* Light) 10
orange marmalade (*Crosse & Blackwell*) 60
Jambalaya dinner mix (*Luzianne*), 1/4 pkg. 200
Java plum, 3 medium, .4 oz. 5
Jelly, 1 tbsp.:
all flavors (*Smucker's*) 50
all flavors except apple and strawberry (*Kraft*) 50
apple or strawberry (*Kraft*) 60
apple with mint (*Crosse & Blackwell*) 50
currant, red (*Crosse & Blackwell*) 60
pepper, mild (*Tabasco*) 60
pepper, spicy (*Tabasco*) 50
Jerk sauce (*World Harbors* Blue Mountain), 2 tbsp. 40
Jerusalem artichoke, sliced, 1/2 cup 57
Jicama, see "Yam bean tuber"

K

FOOD AND MEASURE	CALORIES
Kale:	
fresh, boiled, drained, chopped, ½ cup	21
canned (*Allens/Sunshine*), ½ cup	25
frozen (*Seabrook*), 3 oz.	30
Kale, Scotch, boiled, drained, chopped, ½ cup	18
Kasha, see "Buckwheat groats"	
Ketchup, 1 tbsp.:	
(*Healthy Choice*)	10
(*Heinz*)	15
(*Hunt's/Hunt's* No Salt)	15
KFC, 1 serving:	
Original Recipe chicken:	
breast	360
drumstick	130
thigh	260
wing, whole	150
Colonel's Rotisserie Gold chicken:	
breast and wing	335
breast and wing, without skin and wing (breast meat only)	199
thigh and leg	333
thigh and leg, without skin	217
Extra Tasty Crispy chicken:	
breast	470
drumstick	190
thigh	370
wing, whole	200
Hot & Spicy chicken:	
breast	530
drumstick	190
thigh	370
wing, whole	210
chicken pot pie	730

KFC (cont.)

Crispy Strips, 4 pieces 323
Hot Wings, 6 pieces 471
Kentucky Nuggets, 6 pieces 284
sandwiches:
 chicken 497
 Colonel's chicken 482
 BBQ chicken 256
sides and specials:
 BBQ baked beans 132
 beans, red, and rice 114
 biscuit 200
 coleslaw 114
 corn bread 228
 corn on the cob 222
 garden rice 75
 macaroni and cheese 162
 mashed potatoes with gravy 109
 Mean Greens 52
 potato salad 180
 potato wedges 192

Kidney beans, ½ cup:
dry, boiled 112
canned, red (*Eden* Organic) 100
canned, red (*Hunt's*) 95
canned, red, baked (*B&M*) 170
canned, red, dark (*Allens/East Texas Fair/Trappey's*) 130
canned, red, dark or light (*Stokely*) 120
canned, red, light (*Allens/Trappey's*) 120
canned, red, light, with bacon, chili gravy, or jalapeños
 (*Trappey's*) 110
canned, white (*Progresso* Cannellini) 100

Kielbasa (see also "Polish sausage"):
(*Boar's Head*), 2 oz. 120
(*Jones Dairy Farm* Dinner), 1 link 190

Kiwi:
fresh, 1 large, 3.7 oz. 55
fresh, fuzzless (*Frieda's*), 1 oz. 10
dried (*Sonoma*), 7–8 pieces, 1 oz. 90

Kiwi juice (*After the Fall* Bear Punch), 8 fl. oz. 100
Kiwi-strawberry drink (*Snapple*), 8 fl. oz. 120
Knockwurst, beef (*Boar's Head*), 4 oz. 310
Kohlrabi, boiled, drained, sliced, ½ cup 24
Kumquat, fresh, seeded (*Frieda's*), 1 oz. 18

L

FOOD AND MEASURE	CALORIES
Lamb, choice grade, meat only, 4 oz., except as noted:	
cubed, leg and shoulder, braised or stewed	253
cubed, leg and shoulder, broiled	211
foreshank, braised or stewed, lean with fat	276
foreshank, lean only	212
ground, raw	320
ground, broiled	321
leg, whole, roasted:	
leg, whole, lean with fat	293
leg, whole, lean only	217
leg, shank, lean with fat	255
leg, shank, lean only	204
leg, sirloin, lean with fat	331
leg, sirloin, lean only	231
loin chop, broiled, lean with fat	358
loin chop, broiled, lean with fat, 2.25 oz. (4.2 oz. raw with bone)	201
loin chop, broiled, lean only, 1.6 oz. (4.2 oz. raw with bone and fat)	100
loin, roasted, lean with fat	350
loin, roasted, lean only	229
rib, broiled, lean with fat	409
rib, broiled, lean only	266
shoulder, whole, braised, lean with fat	390
shoulder, whole, braised, lean only	321
shoulder, whole, roasted, lean only	231
Lamb, New Zealand, frozen, meat only, 4 oz.:	
leg, whole, roasted, lean with fat	279
leg, whole, roasted, lean only	205
loin chop, broiled, lean with fat	357
loin chop, broiled, lean only	226
Lamb entree, frozen, curry (*Curry Classics*), 10 oz.	480
Lard, pork, 1 tbsp.	115

Lasagna entree, canned:
(*Hormel/Hormel* Micro Cup), 7.5 oz. 250
(*Libby's Diner*), 7.75 oz. 200
and beef (*Hormel* Micro Cup), 10.5 oz. 359
Italian (*Top Shelf*), 10 oz. 340
Lasagna entree, frozen:
(*Celentano*), 10 oz. 400
(*Celentano* Great Choice), 10 oz. 260
(*Healthy Choice* Roma), 13.5 oz. 390
cheese (*Lean Cuisine* Classic), 11½ oz. 290
cheese, casserole (*Lean Cuisine Lunch Express*), 9½ oz. 270
cheese, with chicken scaloppini (*Lean Cuisine* Cafe
Classics), 10 oz. 290
cheese, four (*Stouffer's*), 10¾ oz. 410
cheese, Italian (*Weight Watchers*), 11 oz. 300
Florentine (*Smart Ones*), 10 oz. 200
garden (*Weight Watchers*), 11 oz. 270
with meat sauce (*Banquet*), 10.5 oz. 290
with meat sauce (*Lean Cuisine*), 10½ oz. 290
with meat sauce (*Marie Callender's*), 7 oz. 370
with meat sauce (*Stouffer's*), 10½ oz. 360
with meat sauce (*Stouffer's Lunch Express*), 10¼ oz. . . 330
with meat sauce (*Swanson*), 10 oz. 410
with meat sauce (*Weight Watchers*), 10.25 oz. 270
with meat sauce, casserole (*Swanson*), 1 pkg. 330
primavera (*Celentano* Great Choice), 10 oz. 240
primavera (*Celentano* Selects), 10 oz. 210
vegetable (*Amy's* Family), 7 oz. 200
vegetable (*Banquet*), 10½ oz. 260
vegetable (*Lean Cuisine*), 10½ oz. 270
vegetable (*Stouffer's*), 10½ oz. 450
vegetable, with cheese (*Amy's*), 9.5 oz. 300
vegetable, cheesy (*Swanson*), 1 pkg. 350
vegetable, tofu (*Amy's*), 9.5 oz. 300
Leek, fresh, raw, trimmed, chopped, ½ cup 32
Lemon, with peel, 2⅛"-diam., 3.9 oz. 22
Lemon juice (*ReaLemon*), 1 tsp. 0
Lemon herb sauce mix (*Knorr*), 1 tbsp. 30
Lemon peel, candied (*S&W*), 58 pieces, 1.1 oz. 80

Lemon sauce (*House of Tsang*), 2 tbsp. 70
Lemonade, 8 fl. oz.:
(*After the Fall*) 90
(*Minute Maid* Regular/Pink) 110
(*Snapple*) 110
(*Veryfine* Chillers) 140
pink (*Snapple*) 120
Lemonade fruit blends, 8 fl. oz.:
all flavors (*R.W. Knudsen/Santa Cruz*) 120
all flavors (*Veryfine* Chillers) 120
all flavors (*Minute Maid*) 120
all flavors, frozen* (*Minute Maid*) 110
cherry (*Snapple*) 130
peach or strawberry (*Snapple*) 120
Lemonade mix* (*Country Time/Country Time* Punch), 8 fl. oz. 70
Lentil:
dry, green or red (*Arrowhead Mills*), ¼ cup 150
cooked, ½ cup 115
Lentil dishes, canned (*Patak's* Moong Dhal), ½ cup . . . 160
Lentil dishes, mix:
hearty, and wild rice (*Spice Islands* Quick Meal), 1 pkg. 190
and herb (*Eastern Traditions*), 2 oz. 160
pilaf (*Casbah*), 1 oz. 100
pilaf (*Near East*), 1 cup* 210
pilaf, almond (*Spice Islands* Quick Meal), 1 pkg. 190
Lentil rice loaf, frozen (*Natural Touch*), 1″ slice 170
Lettuce (see also "Salad blend mix"):
Bibb or Boston, 1 head, 5″ diam. 21
butter (*Dole*), 1 head 21
cos or romaine, 2 inner leaves or ½ cup shredded 4
iceberg, ½ of 6″-diam. head 35
iceberg, precut (*Dole*), 3 oz. 15
leaf, shredded (*Dole*), 1½ cups 12
limestone (*Frieda's*), 1 oz. 4
loose leaf, shredded, ½ cup 5
Lima beans, ½ cup, except as noted:
fresh, mature, baby, boiled 115
fresh, mature, large, boiled 108

canned (*S&W* Butter Beans) 70
canned, baby (*Allens* Butter Beans) 120
canned, green (*Del Monte*) 80
canned, green and white (*Allens*) 110
canned, with bacon, baby green (*Trappey's* Limas) 120
frozen, baby (*Green Giant Harvest Fresh*) 80
frozen, baby, butter sauce (*Green Giant*), 2/3 cup 120
Lime, 1 medium, 2″ diam. 20
Lime drink:
(*After the Fall* Key West), 8 fl. oz. 100
frozen* (*Minute Maid* Limeade) 8 fl. oz. 100
Lime juice (*ReaLime*), 1 tsp. 0
Ling, meat only, baked, broiled, or microwaved, 4 oz. . . 126
Ling cod, meat only, baked, broiled, or microwaved,
4 oz. 124
Linguine, plain:
dry, see also "Pasta"
refrigerated (*Contadina*), 1¼ cup 260
refrigerated, tomato herb (*Contadina*), 1¼ cup 250
Linguine entree mix, with chicken, broccoli (*Noodle Roni*), 1 cup* 370
Liquor, pure distilled, 90 proof, 1 fl. oz. 74
Little Caesars, 1 serving:
Baby Pan!Pan!, 2 squares 616
Crazy Bread, 1 piece 106
Crazy Sauce, 6 oz. 74
Pan!Pan!, cheese only, 1 medium slice 181
Pan!Pan!, pepperoni, 1 medium slice 199
Pizza!Pizza!, cheese only, 1 medium slice 201
Pizza!Pizza!, pepperoni, 1 medium slice 220
salads, individual:
antipasto 176
Caesar 140
Greek 168
tossed 116
dressings, 1.5 oz.:
blue cheese 160
Caesar 255
French 166

Little Caesars*, dressings, 1.5 oz. *(cont.)
Greek 268
Italian 200
Italian, fat free 15
ranch 221
1000 Island 183
sandwiches, cold:
ham and cheese 728
Italian 740
veggie 647
sandwiches, hot:
Cheeser 822
Meatsa 1036
pepperoni 899
supreme 894

Liver:
beef, pan fried, 4 oz. 246
chicken, simmered, chopped, 1 cup 219
lamb, pan fried, 4 oz. 270
pork, braised, 4 oz. 187
turkey, simmered, chopped, 1 cup 237
veal (calves), braised, 4 oz. 187

Liver cheese (*Oscar Mayer*), 1.3-oz. slice 120

Liverwurst (see also "Braunschweiger"):
(*Boar's Head* Strassburger/Smoked), 2 oz. 170
(*Underwood*), 2 oz. 160
spread (*Hormel*), 2 oz. 130

Lobster, northern, meat only, boiled or steamed, 1 cup, 5.1 oz. 142

"Lobster," imitation, frozen or refrigerated:
chunks (*Captain Jac Lobster Tasties*), ½ cup, 3 oz. 90
tail style (*Captain Jac Lobster Tasties*), 4-oz. tail 100

Lobster, spiny, see "Spiny lobster"

Lobster sauce, rock, canned (*Progresso*), ½ cup 100

Loganberry, fresh, 1 cup 89

Long John Silver's:
chicken and seafood:
chicken, batter-dipped, 2-oz. piece 120
chicken, *Flavorbaked,* 2.6-oz. piece 110

chicken, popcorn, 3.3 oz. 250
clams, 3 oz. 300
fish, batter-dipped, 3-oz. piece 170
fish, *Flavorbaked,* 2.3-oz. piece 90
fish, popcorn, 3.6 oz. 290
shrimp, batter-dipped, .4-oz. piece 35
shrimp, popcorn, 3.3 oz. 280

sandwiches:

chicken, *Flavorbaked,* 5.8 oz. 290
fish, batter-dipped, without sauce, 5.4 oz. 320
fish, *Flavorbaked,* 6 oz. 320
Ultimate Fish, 6.4 oz. 430

side dishes:

cheese sticks, 1.6 oz. 160
coleslaw, 3.4 oz. 140
corn cobbette, 3.3 oz. 140
corn cobbette, without butter, 3.1 oz. 80
french fries, 3 oz. 250
green beans, 3.5 oz. 30
hush puppy, .8-oz. piece 60
potato, baked, 8 oz. 210
rice pilaf, 3 oz. 140
salad, side, 4.3 oz. 25

condiments and dressings:

French dressing, fat free, 1.5 oz. 50
honey mustard sauce, .4 oz. 20
Italian dressing, 1 oz. 130
malt vinegar, .3 oz. 0
margarine, .2 oz. 35
ranch dressing, 1 oz. 170
ranch dressing, fat free, 1.5 oz. 50
shrimp sauce, .4 oz. 15
sour cream, 1 oz. 60
sweet 'n' sour sauce, .4 oz. 20
tartar sauce, .4 oz. 35
Thousand Island dressing, 1 oz. 110

Loquat (*Frieda's*), 3.5 oz. 48
Lotus root, boiled, drained, 4 oz. 75
Lox, see "Salmon, smoked"

Luncheon meat (see also specific listings):
loaf, spiced (*Oscar Mayer*), 1-oz. slice 70
canned (*Spam/Spam* Less Salt), 2 oz. 170
canned, light (*Spam* Lite), 2 oz. 110
canned, spread (*Spam*), 2 oz. 100
Lupin, boiled, ½ cup 98
Lupini beans, in jars (*Canto*), ¼ cup 30
Lychees:
shelled, raw, peeled (*Frieda's*), 1 oz. 18
dried, 1 oz. 79

M

FOOD AND MEASURE **CALORIES**

Macadamia nut, shelled:
dried, 1 cup 940
oil-roasted, 1 oz. 204
Macaroni (see also "Pasta"):
uncooked, 2 oz. 211
cooked, elbow, 1 cup 197
cooked, small shells, 1 cup 162
cooked, spirals, 1 cup 189
cooked, vegetable (tri-color), 4 oz. 145
cooked, whole wheat, 4 oz. 141
Macaroni dinner, and cheese, frozen (*Swanson* Budget),
1 pkg. 320
Macaroni entree, canned:
and beef (*Libby's Diner*), 7.75 oz. 220
and cheese (*Chef Boyardee* Bowl), 7.5 oz. 160
and cheese (*Hormel* Micro Cup), 7.5 oz. 260
and cheese (*Libby's Diner*), 7.75 oz. 320
Macaroni entree, frozen:
and beef (*Lean Cuisine*), 10 oz. 280
and beef (*Stouffer's*), 11½ oz. 420
and beef casserole (*Swanson*), 1 pkg. 270
broccoli (*Swanson Mac & More*),
1 pkg. 220
and cheese (*Amy's*), 9 oz. 450
and cheese (*Lean Cuisine*), 9 oz. 270
and cheese (*Stouffer's*), ½ of 12-oz. pkg. 330
and cheese (*Swanson* Entree), 1 pkg. 280
and cheese (*Swanson* Entree), 1 cup 260
and cheese (*Swanson Mac & More* Classic), 1 pkg. . . . 240
and cheese, three-cheese casserole (*Swanson*), 1 pkg. . . 400
and cheese, white cheddar (*Swanson Mac & More*), 1
pkg. 200
and cheese, salsa (*Swanson Mac & More*), 1 pkg. 210

Macaroni entree, frozen ***(cont.)***
Italiano (*Swanson Mac & More*), 1 pkg. or pie 180
soy cheeze (*Amy's*), 9 oz. 360
Macaroni entree mix, dry, except as noted:
(*Creamette*), 1/3 pkg. 250
and cheese, cheddar (*Golden Grain*), 1 cup* 340
and cheese, rotini, with broccoli (*Velveeta*), 4.5 oz. 400
and cheese, shells, plain or with bacon (*Velveeta* Original), 4 oz. 360
and cheese, shells, with salsa (*Velveeta* Original), 4 oz. 380
and cheese, three cheese (*Knorr* Cup), 1 pkg. 240
Macaroni and cheese, see "Macaroni dinner" and "Macaroni entree"
Mackerel, meat only:
Atlantic, baked, broiled, or microwaved, 4 oz. 297
king, baked, broiled, or microwaved, 4 oz. 152
Pacific and jack, baked, broiled, or microwaved, 4 oz. . . 228
Spanish, baked, broiled, or microwaved, 4 oz. 179
smoked (*Spence & Co.*), 2 oz. 180
Mackerel, canned, drained:
jack, 4 oz. 177
skinless, boneless (*Reese*), 4.375-oz. can 240
Mahi mahi:
fresh, see "Dolphinfish"
frozen, fillet (*Peter Pan*), 4 oz. 100
Malt cooler (*Bartles & Jaymes*), 12-oz. bottle:
berry, peach, or strawberry 210
black cherry or red sangria 200
Fuzzy Navel or tropical 230
iced tea, Long Island 250
Mai Tai 240
Margarita 260
original 190
piña colada 270
Malted milk powder:
natural (*Kraft*), 3 tbsp. 80
chocolate (*Kraft*), 3 tbsp. 90
Mammy apple, peeled, seeded, 1 oz. 14
Mango:

fresh, peeled, sliced, ½ cup 54
dried (*Sonoma*), 8 pieces, 2 oz. 180
frozen, chunks (*Goya*), ⅓ pkg. 100
Mango drink, 8 fl. oz.:
(*Snapple* Madness) 110
(*Tree Top* More Mango) 120
tangerine (*Veryfine* Arctic) 110
Mango juice (*After the Fall* Montage), 8 fl. oz. 110
Mango nectar (*Libby's/Kern's*), 8 fl. oz. 150
Mango-orange nectar (*Kern's*), 8 fl. oz. 140
Mango-peach juice (*R.W. Knudsen*), 8 fl. oz. 120
Manhattan mixer, bottled (*Holland House*), 2 fl. oz. 60
Manicotti, frozen, 2 pieces:
(*Celentano*), 7 oz. 410
mini (*Celentano*), 4.8 oz. 110
Manicotti entree, frozen:
cheese (*Celentano*), 10 oz. 450
cheese (*Celentano* Great Choice), 10 oz. 250
cheese (*Celentano* Value Pack), 2 pieces, 8 oz. 320
cheese (*Stouffer's*), 9 oz. 340
cheese (*Weight Watchers*), 9.25 oz. 260
cheese, three (*Healthy Choice*), 11 oz. 310
Florentine (*Celentano*), 10 oz. 220
Florentine (*Celentano* Great Choice), 10 oz. 210
Maple syrup (*Cary's/Maple Orchards/MacDonald's*),
¼ cup 210
Margarine, 1 tbsp., except as noted:
(*Mazola/Mazola* Unsalted) 100
(*Mazola* Light) 50
(*Smart Beat* Nonfat) 10
(*Smart Beat* Super Light/Trans Fat Free) 20
(*Smart Beat* Unsalted) 25
soft (*Parkay* Tub) 100
spread (*Mazola* Light) 50
squeeze (*Parkay*) 80
whipped (*Parkay* Tub) 70
Margarita mixer:
bottled (*Holland House*), 4 fl. oz. 130
bottled, strawberry (*Holland House*), 3.5 fl. oz. 150

frozen* (*Bacardi*), 8 fl. oz. 90
Marinade (see also "Stir-fry sauce" and specific listings):
(*House of Tsang* Classic), ½ tbsp. 15
(*House of Tsang Mandarin*), 1 tbsp. 25
Hawaiian (*Lawry's*), 1 tbsp. 20
lemon butter dill, seafood (*Ken's Steak House*). 1 tbsp. . . 50
lemon pepper or red wine (*Lawry's*), 1 tbsp. 10
and stir-fry sauce (*Mary Rose* Sari), 1 tbsp. 5
Marinade seasoning mix, meat (*Lawry's* Carne Asada), 1 tsp. 5
Marrow squash, raw, trimmed, 1 oz. 4
Marshmallow topping, all varieties (*Marshmallow Fluff*), 2 tbsp. 60
Mayonnaise, 1 tbsp.:
(*Hellmann's/Best Foods* Real) 100
(*Hellmann's/Best Foods* Light) 50
(*Hellmann's/Best Foods* Low Fat) 25
dressing (*Miracle Whip* Salad) 70
dressing (*Miracle Whip Free*) 15
dressing (*Miracle Whip Light*) 40
McDonald's 1 serving:
breakfast biscuit:
plain 260
bacon, egg, and cheese 440
sausage 430
sausage and egg 520
breakfast burrito 320
breakfast dishes:
eggs, scrambled, 2 170
hash browns 130
hotcakes, plain 310
hotcakes, with syrup and margarine 580
sausage 170
breakfast muffin:
English 140
Egg McMuffin 290
Sausage McMuffin 360
Sausage McMuffin, with egg 440

danish and muffins:
- apple bran muffin 170
- apple danish 360
- cheese danish 410
- cinnamon-raisin danish 430
- raspberry danish 400

sandwiches:
- *Arch Deluxe* 570
- *Arch Deluxe,* with bacon 610
- *Big Mac* 530
- cheeseburger 320
- *Filet-O-Fish* 360
- hamburger 270
- *McChicken* 510
- *McGrilled Chicken Classic* 260
- *Quarter Pounder* 420
- *Quarter Pounder,* with cheese 530

Chicken McNuggets:
- 4 pieces 190
- 6 pieces 290
- 9 pieces 430

McNuggets sauce, 1 pkt.:
- barbecue or honey 45
- honey mustard or sweet and sour 50
- hot mustard 60

french fries:
- small 210
- large 450
- *Super Size* 540

salads:
- chicken, fajita 160
- garden 80

salad bacon bits, 1 pkg. 15

salad croutons, 1 pkg. 50

salad dressing, 1 pkg.:
- blue cheese 190
- ranch 230
- red French, reduced calorie 160
- Thousand Island 190

McDonald's*, salad dressing *(cont.)
vinaigrette, lite 50
desserts and shakes:
baked apple pie 260
McDonaldland Cookies, 1 pkg. 260
shake, small, all flavors 340
sundae, hot fudge 290
yogurt, frozen, lowfat:
cone, vanilla 120
hot caramel sundae 310
strawberry sundae 240
Meat, see specific listings
Meat, canned:
potted (*Hormel*), 2 oz. 100
potted or deviled (*Libby's*), 3 oz. 160
"Meat," ground, frozen (*Morningstar Farms* Ground
Meatless), ½ cup 60
Meat loaf dinner, frozen:
(*Banquet*), 19 oz. 650
(*Healthy Choice*), 12 oz. 320
(*Marie Callender's*), 14 oz. 540
(*Swanson*), 1 pkg. 380
(*Swanson* Budget), 1 pkg. 330
(*Swanson Hungry Man*), 1 pkg. 610
Meat loaf entree, frozen:
(*Banquet* Homestyle), 9.5 oz. 280
with whipped potato (*Stouffer's* Homestyle), 9⅞ oz. . . . 390
tomato sauce with (*Morton*), 9 oz. 250
with sauce and vegetables (*Swanson*), 1 pkg. 260
with whipped potato (*Lean Cuisine*), 9⅜ oz. 250
"Meat" loaf mix, vegetarian (*Natural Touch*), ¼ cup . . . 100
Meat loaf seasoning mix:
(*Durkee* Pouch), 1/9 pkt. 20
(*Durkee/French's* Roasting Bag), ⅛ pkg. 15
(*Lawry's*), 1 tbsp. 35
Meat spread, see "Sandwich spread"
Meatball entree (see also "Spaghetti entree"), frozen:
kofta curry (*Deep*), 5 oz. 245
Swedish (*Healthy Choice*), 11.1 oz. 320

Swedish (*Stouffer's*), 9¼ oz. 440
Swedish (*Weight Watchers*), 9 oz. 280
Swedish, with broccoli (*Stouffer's Lunch Express*), 10⅜ oz. 360
Swedish, with pasta (*Lean Cuisine*), 9⅛ oz. 290
Swedish, with pasta (*Stouffer's Lunch Express*), 10¼ oz. 530
Meatball seasoning mix, Italian (*Durkee* Pouch), ⅕ pkt. . 20
Meatball stew, canned (*Dinty Moore*), 1 cup 270
Melon balls, frozen, cantaloupe and honeydew, ½ cup 2
Melon drink blend (*Tree Top* Wonder Melon), 8 fl. oz. . . 120
Menudo, canned (*Goya*), 1 cup 200
Mesquite sauce, cooking and marinade (*S&W*), 1 tbsp. 10
Mexican beans (see also "Chili beans"), canned, ½ cup:
(*Allens/Brown Beauty*) 120
(*Chi-Chi's* Ranchero) 100
(*Stokely* Red) 110
with jalapeños (*Trappey's* Mexi-Beans) 130
Mexican dinner (see also specific listings), frozen:
(*Patio*), 13.25 oz. 430
(*Patio* Fiesta), 12 oz. 340
(*Patio* Ranchera), 13 oz. 410
Mexican style (*Swanson Hungry Man*), 1 pkg. 780
Mexican style, combination (*Swanson*), 1 pkg. 470
Mexican seasoning (*Chi-Chi's* Mix), 1 tsp. 10
Milk, 8 fl. oz.:
buttermilk, cultured 99
whole, 3.3% fat 150
lowfat, 2% fat 121
lowfat, 2%, protein fortified 137
lowfat, 1% fat 102
lowfat, 1%, protein fortified 119
skim 86
Milk, canned:
condensed, sweet (*Carnation*), 2 tbsp. 130
evaporated (*Carnation*), 2 tbsp. 40
evaporated, lowfat or skim (*Carnation*), 2 tbsp. 25
Milk, chocolate, see "Chocolate milk"
Milk, dry:
buttermilk, sweet cream, 1 tbsp. 25

whole, 1 oz. 141
nonfat (*Carnation*), ⅓ cup 80
Milk, goat's, 1 cup 168
"Milk," nondairy (see also "Soy beverage"), 8 fl. oz.:
(*Rice Dream* Original) 120
chocolate (*Rice Dream*) 160
vanilla (*Rice Dream*) 130
Milk, sheep's, 1 cup 264
Milkfish, meat only, baked, broiled, or microwaved, 4 oz. 215
Millet, cooked, 4 oz. 135
Mint sauce (*Crosse & Blackwell*), 1 tsp. 5
Miso, soy (*Eden* Hacho), 1 tbsp. 35
Mocha drink, chilled (*Nestlé Mocha Cooler*), 1 cup 170
Molasses, blackstrap (*New Morning*), 1 tbsp. 60
Monkfish, meat only, baked, broiled, or microwaved, 4 oz. 110
Mortadella, 2 oz.:
(*Boar's Head Cinghiale*) 160
with pistachios (*Boar's Head Cinghiale*) 170
Muffin, 1 piece, except as noted:
(*Arnold Bran'nola*) 130
(*Arnold* Extra Crisp) 120
all flavors except blueberry, mini (*Hostess*), 5 pieces . . . 260
apple, blueberry, or corn (*Awrey's*), 1.5 oz. 130
banana nut (*Awrey's* Grande), 4 oz. 400
blueberry (*Awrey's* Grande), 4 oz. 340
blueberry, mini (*Hostess*), 5 pieces 240
carrot, raisin (*Awrey's* Grande), 4 oz. 360
cheese streusel (*Awrey's* Grande), 4 oz. 380
chocolate chocolate chip (*Awrey's* Grande), 4 oz. 460
cranberry nut (*Awrey's*), 1.5 oz. 120
English (*Awrey's*) 140
English, regular, oat bran, or sourdough (*Thomas'*) 120
English, blueberry, cranberry, or raisin (*Thomas'*) 140
English, honey wheat (*Thomas'*) 110
English, sandwich size (*Thomas'* 4 Pack) 190
lemon poppyseed (*Awrey's*), 1.5 oz. 170
raisin (*Arnold*) 150
raisin bran (*Awrey's*), 1.5 oz. 110

raisin bran (*Awrey's* Grande), 4 oz. 350
sourdough (*Arnold*) 120
Muffin, frozen or refrigerated, 1 piece:
apple oatmeal (*Pepperidge Farm Wholesome Choice*) . . . 160
blueberry (*Pepperidge Farm Wholesome Choice*) 140
English (*Thomas'*) 120
English, honey wheat (*Thomas'*) 110
raisin bran or corn (*Pepperidge Farm Wholesome Choice*) 150
Mulberries, ½ cup 31
Mullet, striped, meat only, baked, broiled, or microwaved, 4 oz. 170
Mung beans:
dry (*Arrowhead Mills*), ¼ cup 160
boiled, ½ cup 107
Mung beans, sprouted, fresh, raw (*Jonathan's*), 1 cup . . . 30
Mushroom:
fresh, raw, pieces, ½ cup 9
fresh, boiled, drained, pieces, ½ cup 21
canned, all varieties, except with garlic (*B in B*), 4¼-oz. can 30
canned, with garlic, sliced (*B in B*), 4¼-oz. can 35
enoki, 1 large, 4⅛" long 2
Japanese honey, trimmed (*Frieda's*), 1 oz. 9
oyster, fresh or dried (*Frieda's*), 1 oz. 7
portobello, fresh (*Frieda's*), 1 oz. 8
portobello, dried (*Frieda's*), ½ oz. 13
shiitake, cooked, 4 medium or ½-cup pieces 40
shiitake, dried, 4 medium, .5 oz. 44
Mushroom gravy, ¼ cup:
country or with wine (*Pepperidge Farm*), ¼ cup 30
creamy or regular (*Franco-American*), ¼ cup 20
mix*, brown (*Durkee*), ¼ cup 15
mix, hunter (*Knorr*), 1 tbsp. 25
Mushroom sauce (*House of Tsang*), 1 tbsp. 10
Mushroom sauce mix (*Knorr*), ⅕ pkg., 2 tsp. 20
Mussel, blue, meat only, boiled or steamed, 4 oz. 195
Mustard, prepared, 1 tsp., except as noted:
brown (*Gulden's* Spicy) 0

Mustard ***(cont.)***
Chinese (*House of Tsang*), 1 pkt. 15
Dijon (*Roland* Extra Strong) 10
hot or sharp and creamy (*Nance's*) 15
Mustard blend (*Hellmann's/Best Foods Dijonnaise*),
1 tsp. 5
Mustard greens:
fresh, raw, chopped, 1 oz. or ½ cup 7
fresh, chopped, boiled, drained, ½ cup 11
canned (*Allens/Sunshine*), ½ cup 30
frozen, chopped (*Seabrook*), 3 oz. 30
Mustard spinach, ½ cup:
fresh, raw, chopped 17
fresh, chopped, boiled 14

N

FOOD AND MEASURE	CALORIES
Natto, ½ cup	187
Navy beans, ½ cup:	
fresh, boiled	129
canned (*Stokely*)	110
canned, with bacon or bacon and jalapeños (*Trappey's*)	110
Navy beans, sprouted, raw, ½ cup	35
Nectarine, fresh:	
1 medium, 2½" diam.	67
sliced, ½ cup	34
New Zealand spinach, chopped:	
raw, 1 oz. or ½ cup	4
boiled, drained, ½ cup	11
Newburg sauce mix (*Knorr*), ⅓ pkg.	30
Noodle:	
Chinese (*Nasoya*), 1 cup, 2.75 oz.	210
Chinese, cellophane or long rice, dry, 2 oz.	199
Chinese, chow mein (*La Choy*), ½ cup	140
Chinese, crispy, wide (*La Choy*), ½ cup	150
Chinese, egg, dried (*House of Tsang*), 2 oz.	200
Chinese, rice (*La Choy*), ½ cup	120
egg, uncooked, all varieties (*Creamette/Goodman's*), 2 oz.	220
egg, uncooked, bow ties (*Mueller's*), 2 oz.	220
egg, cooked, 1 cup	212
Japanese (*Nasoya*), 1 cup, 2.75 oz.	210
Japanese, soba, dry, 2 oz.	192
Japanese, soba, cooked, 1 cup	113
Japanese, somen, dry, 2 oz.	203
Japanese, somen, cooked, 1 cup	230
Japanese, spinach (*Nasoya*), 1 cup, 2.75 oz.	210
Japanese, udon, dry, 2 oz.	159
Japanese, udon, cooked, 4 oz.	115

Noodle dishes, mix, dry, ½ pkg., except as noted:
Alfredo (*Lipton* Noodles & Sauce) 250
Alfredo, carbonara or broccoli (*Lipton* Noodles & Sauce) 260
beef (*Lipton* Noodles & Sauce) 220
butter or Romanoff (*Lipton* Noodles & Sauce) 260
butter and herb (*Lipton* Noodles & Sauce) 250
with cheddar (*Master-A-Meal*), ⅕ pkg. 180
cheddar-bacon or chicken (*Lipton* Noodles & Sauce) . . . 230
cheese or Parmesan (*Lipton* Noodles & Sauce) 250
chicken, broccoli or tetrazzini (*Lipton* Noodles & Sauce) 220
chicken, creamy (*Lipton* Noodles & Sauce) 230
Oriental (*Knorr* Cup), 1 pkg. 210
sour cream and chive (*Lipton* Noodles & Sauce) 260
Stroganoff (*Lipton* Noodles & Sauce) 210

Noodle entree, canned:
with beef (*Hunt's* Homestyle), 1 cup 150
with beef (*La Choy* Bi-Pack), 1 cup 150
with chicken (*Hormel* Micro Cup), 7.5 oz. 200
with chicken (*La Choy* Bi-Pack), 1 cup 160
with chicken, cacciatore or regular (*Hunt's* Homestyle), 1 cup 175
with chicken and mushrooms (*Hunt's* Homestyle), 1 cup 200
sweet and sour, with chicken (*La Choy* Entree), 1 cup . . 260
with vegetables (*La Choy* Entree), 1 cup 130
with vegetables and beef or chicken (*La Choy* Entree), 1 cup 160

Noodle entree, frozen:
and beef, with gravy (*Banquet* Family), 1 cup 140
and chicken (*Banquet* Bake at Home), 8-oz. cup 210
and chicken, escalloped (*Marie Callender's*), 6.5 oz. 270
kung pao, and vegetables (*Weight Watchers*), 10 oz. . . . 260
Romanoff (*Stouffer's*), 12 oz. 490

Nut topping (see also specific listings) (*Planters*), 2 tbsp. 100

Nuts, see specific listings

Nuts, mixed, salted or unsalted, 1 oz.:
dry-roasted (*Planters*) 170
honey-roasted (*Planters*) 140

oil-roasted:
(*Planters/Planters* Deluxe/*Planters* Lightly Salted/
Unsalted) 170
cashews, with almonds/macadamias or pecans
(*Planters* Select) 170
sesame (*Planters*) 150
tamari-roasted (*Eden*) 170

O

FOOD AND MEASURE	CALORIES
Oat (see also "Cereal"):	
whole grain, 1 oz.	110
flakes, rolled (*Arrowhead Mills*), 1/3 cup	130
rolled or oatmeal, cooked, 1 cup	145
steel cut (*Arrowhead Mills*), 1/4 cup	170
Oat bran, dry (*Arrowhead Mills*), 1/3 cup	150
Oat flour (*Arrowhead Mills*), 1/3 cup	120
Oat groats (*Arrowhead Mills*), 1/4 cup	160
Ocean perch, meat only, baked, broiled, or microwaved, 4 oz.	137
Ocean perch, frozen:	
(*Van de Kamp's* Natural), 4 oz.	130
battered (*Gorton's* Crispy), 2 pieces	300
Octopus, meat only, boiled or steamed, 4 oz.	186
Octopus, canned:	
(*Goya*), 1/4 cup	140
in garlic sauce or olive oil (*Goya*), 1/4 cup	150
Oheloberry, 1/2 cup	20
Oil, 1 tbsp., except as noted:	
all varieties and blends (*Wesson*)	122
almond, canola, cocoa butter, corn, cottonseed, hazelnut, nutmeg butter, oat, olive, palm, palm kernel, peanut, poppyseed, safflower, sesame, soybean, sunflower, vegetable, or walnut	120
avocado or mustard	124
butter oil	112
coconut	117
cod liver or herring	123
Oriental cooking, sesame or wok (*House of Tsang*), 1 tsp.	45
popcorn, popping and topping (*Orville Redenbacher*)	120
salmon or sardine	123
Oil substitute (*Baking Healthy*), 1 tbsp.	30

Okra, ½ cup, except as noted:
fresh, boiled drained, sliced 25
canned, cut or with tomatoes (*Allens/Trappey's*) 25
canned, Creole gumbo (*Trappey's*) 35
frozen, whole (*Seabrook*), 9 pods, 3 oz. 25
Old-fashioned drink mixer, bottled (*Holland House*), 2 fl. oz. 80
Old-fashioned loaf (*Oscar Mayer*), 1-oz. slice 60
Olive, pickled:
Alfonso (*Krinos*), ½ oz. 30
Calamata (*Krinos*), 3 olives, ½ oz. 45
green, with pits, 10 large 45
green, pitted, 1 oz. 33
green, cracked (*Krinos*), ½ oz. 20
green, queen (*S&W*), 2 olives 20
green, stuffed, Manzanilla (*S&W*), 3 olives 25
green, stuffed, queen (*S&W*, 4¾ oz.), 2 olives 15
ripe, pitted (*Vlasic*), 6 small or 4 large 25
ripe, pitted, Spanish (*Vlasic*), 8 small 20
ripe, with pits (*S&W*), 1 super colossal 15
ripe, oil-cured (*Progresso*), 6 olives 80
ripe, Greek style, 10 medium 65
ripe, Greek style (*Zorba*), 1.7-oz. olive 60
royal (*Krinos*), ½ oz. 30
Olive loaf (*Boar's Head*), 2 oz. 130
Olive salad, drained (*Progresso*), 2 tbsp. 25
Onion, mature:
fresh or stored, raw, 1 oz. 11
fresh or stored, raw, chopped, ½ cup 30
fresh or stored, raw, chopped, 1 tbsp. 4
fresh or stored, boiled, drained, chopped, ½ cup 47
canned or in jars:
whole (*Green Giant*), ½ cup 35
whole (*S&W*), ½ cup 40
cocktail (*Crosse & Blackwell*), 1 tbsp. 5
cocktail (*S&W* 4 oz.), 12 pieces, 1.1 oz. 5
sweet, in sauce (*Boar's Head* Vidalia), 1 tbsp. 10
wild, marinated, (*Krinos* Volvi), 1 oz. 15
frozen, chopped (*Ore-Ida*), ¾ cup 25

Onion ***(cont.)***
frozen rings, see "Onion rings"
Onion, dried, flakes, 1 tbsp. 16
Onion, green, raw, trimmed, with top, chopped, 1 tbsp. 2
Onion, Welsh, trimmed, 1 oz. 10
Onion dip, French, 2 tbsp.:
(*Heluva* Good) 50
(*Nalley's*) 100
(*Ruffles*) 70
sour cream and (*Lay's*) 40
Onion dip mix, and chive (*Knorr*), ½ tsp. 5
Onion gravy, ¼ cup:
roasted, and garlic (*Pepperidge Farm*) 25
zesty (*Heinz* Home Style) 20
mix* (*Durkee*) 10
mix*, brown, Lyonnaise (*Knorr*) 20
Onion powder (*Tone's*), ¼ tsp. 5
Onion rings, frozen:
(*Mrs. Paul's* Old Fashioned), 7 rings 230
(*Ore-Ida* Classic/Gourmet), 4 rings 220
Onion salt (*Tone's*), 1 tsp. 1
Onion sprouts (*Jonathan's*), 1 cup 30
Opossum, meat only, roasted, 4 oz. 251
Orange:
California navel, 2⅞"-diam. orange 65
California Valencia, 2⅝"-diam. orange 59
Florida, 2¾"-diam. orange 70
Orange drink, 8 fl. oz.:
(Bright and Early) 120
orangeade (*Snapple*) 120
Orange drink blends, 8 fl. oz.:
guava nectar (*Kern's*) 150
pineapple (*Lincoln*) 130
punch (*Minute Maid*) 120
Orange drink mix* (Tang), 8 fl. oz. 100
Orange juice, 8 fl. oz., except as noted:
fresh, 6 fl. oz. 83
chilled or frozen*, all varieties, except calcium rich
(*Minute Maid* Premium) 110

chilled or frozen*, calcium rich (*Minute Maid* Premium) 120
Orange juice blends, 8 fl. oz.:
kiwi–passion fruit or pineapple (*Tropicana* Tropics) 100
mango (*R.W. Knudsen*) 120
peach-mango (*Tropicana* Tropics) 110
punch (*Juicy Juice*) 120
punch (*Veryfine* Juice-Ups) 140
Orange peel, candied (*S&W*), 58 pieces, 1.1 oz. 80
Orange sauce, Mandarin (*Ka-Me*), 2 tbsp. 80
Oriental 5-spice (*Tone's*), 1 tsp. 9
Oriental sauce (see also "Stir-fry sauce" and specific listings):
(*House of Tsang* Chow Chow/*House of Tsang*Hunan), 1 tsp. 5
(*House of Tsang* Imperial), 1 tbsp. 25
(*House of Tsang* Namasu), 1 tsp. 10
brown, spicy (*House of Tsang*), 1 tsp. 15
Oyster, meat only:
Eastern, wild, raw, 6 medium, 3 oz. 57
Eastern, wild, baked, broiled, or microwaved, 4 oz. 82
Eastern, wild, steamed or poached, 4 oz. 155
Eastern, farmed, raw, 4 oz. 67
Eastern, farmed, baked, broiled, or microwaved, 4 oz. . . . 90
Pacific, raw, 4 oz. 93
Pacific, boiled or steamed, 4 oz. 185
Oyster, canned:
Eastern, wild, with liquid, 1 cup 170
whole (*S&W*), 2 oz. 70
smoked (*S&W*), 2 oz. 100
Oyster plant, see "Salsify"
Oyster and shrimp sauce (*TryMe* Caribbean Clipper), 1 tsp. 10
Oyster stew, see "Soup"

P–Q

FOOD AND MEASURE	CALORIES
Palm, hearts of, in jars (*Haddon House*), 4.5 oz.	20
Pancake, frozen, 3 pieces:	
(*Aunt Jemima* Original)	200
(*Downyflake*)	270
original or buttermilk (*Hungry Jack* Microwave)	240
Pancake breakfast, frozen, 1 pkg.:	
with bacon (*Swanson Great Starts*)	400
with sausage (*Swanson Great Starts*)	490
silver dollar, eggs and (*Swanson Great Starts*)	250
silver dollar, and sausage (*Swanson Great Starts*)	340
Pancake mix, 1/3 cup dry, except as noted:	
(*Aunt Jemima* Original)	150
(*Aunt Jemima* Complete/Buttermilk Complete)	190
(*Hungry Jack* Original/*Hungry Jack Hungry Lights* Complete)	150
(*Hungry Jack* Premeasured), 1/2 pkt.	200
buckwheat (*Arrowhead Mills*)	140
buckwheat (*Aunt Jemima*), 1/4 cup	120
buttermilk (*Arrowhead Mills*), 1/4 cup	120
buttermilk (*Aunt Jemima* Complete Reduced Calorie)	140
buttermilk (*Hungry Jack/Hungry Jack* Complete)	160
gluten-free or kamut (*Arrowhead Mills*), 1/4 cup	130
oat bran or wild rice (*Arrowhead Mills*)	140
whole wheat (*Aunt Jemima*), 1/4 cup	130
Pancake syrup (see also "Maple syrup"), 1/4 cup:	
all varieties (*Hungry Jack*)	210
all varieties (*Hungry Jack* Lite)	100
Pancreas:	
beef, braised, 4 oz.	307
veal, braised, 4 oz.	290
Papaya:	
fresh, peeled (*Frieda's*), 1 oz.	11
frozen, slices (*Goya*), 1/3 pkg.	50

Papaya drink, 8 fl. oz., except as noted:
(*Farmer's Market*) 130
colada (*Snapple*) 120
nectar (*Libby's/Kern's*), 11.5 fl. oz. 210
punch (*Lincoln*) 130
Papaya juice (*After the Fall* Pele's), 8 fl. oz. 100
Pappadums:
(*Patak's*), 3 pieces, 1 oz. 80
snack crisps (*Tamarind Tree*), 30 pieces, 1 oz. 140
Parsley, fresh, chopped, ½ cup 11
Parsnip, boiled, drained, sliced, ½ cup 63
Passion fruit, purple (*Frieda's*), 3.5 oz. 90
Passion fruit juice, bottled (*Snapple* Supreme), 10 fl. oz. 160
Passion fruit–mango drink (*Heinke's*), 8 fl. oz. 130
Pasta, dry (see also "Macaroni" and specific listings):
uncooked, all varieties (*Creamette/Prince*) 210
uncooked, all varieties (*Delverde*), 2 oz. 200
uncooked, with egg, all varieties (*Herb's*), 2 oz. 220
cooked, plain, 1 cup 197
cooked, corn, 1 cup 176
cooked, spinach, 1 cup 183
cooked, whole wheat, 1 cup 174
Pasta, refrigerated (see also specific listings), uncooked,
2 oz. 164
Pasta dinner, see specific listings
Pasta dishes, frozen (see also "Pasta entree, frozen"):
Alfredo (*Green Giant Pasta Accents*), 2 cups 210
cheddar, creamy (*Green Giant Pasta Accents*), 2⅓ cup . . 250
cheddar, white (*Green Giant Pasta Accents*), 1¾ cups . . 300
Florentine (*Green Giant Pasta Accents*), 2 cups 310
garden herb seasoning (*Green Giant Pasta Accents*),
2 cups 230
garlic seasoning (*Green Giant Pasta Accents*), 2 cups . . 260
primavera (*Green Giant Pasta Accents*), 2¼ cups 320
Pasta dishes, mix (see also specific listings), dry,
except as noted:
cheese, cheddar broccoli (*Lipton* Pasta & Sauce), ½ pkg. 260
chicken, primavera (*Lipton* Pasta & Sauce), ½ pkg. 220
garlic, creamy, corkscrews (*Noodle Roni*), 1 cup* 420

Pasta dishes, mix *(cont.)*
primavera (*Knorr* Cup), 1 pkg. 210
primavera (*Lipton* Pasta & Sauce), ½ pkg. 240
salad, Caesar, creamy (*Kraft*), 2.5 oz. 350
salad, garden primavera (*Kraft*), 2.5 oz. 280
salad, Parmesan peppercorn or ranch with bacon (*Kraft*), 2.5 oz. 360
tomato, creamy, twists (*Knorr* Cup), 1 pkg. 230

Pasta entree, canned (see also specific listings):
spirals, and chicken (*Libby's Diner*), 7.75 oz. 130
twists, with meat sauce (*Franco-American*), 1 cup 250

Pasta entree, frozen (see also specific pasta listings):
cheddar bake with (*Lean Cuisine*), 9 oz. 220
cheddar and broccoli (*Banquet*), 10.5 oz. 350
and chicken marinara (*Lean Cuisine Lunch Express*), 9⅛ oz. 270
marinara twist (*Lean Cuisine*), 10 oz. 240
primavera, with chicken (*Marie Callender's*), 1 cup 310
rings (*Swanson Fun Feast* Razzlin'), 1 pkg. 380
sausage and peppers (*Banquet*), 10.5 oz. 340
and spinach Romano (*Weight Watchers*), 10.4 oz. 240
with tomato basil sauce (*Weight Watchers*), 9.6 oz. 260
and tuna casserole (*Lean Cuisine Lunch Express*), 9⅝ oz. 280
and turkey Dijon (*Lean Cuisine Lunch Express*), 9⅞ oz. 270
vegetable Italiano (*Healthy Choice*), 10 oz. 240

Pasta sauce, tomato (see also specific sauce listings), ½ cup:
(*Prego*) 140
(*Prego Extra Chunky* Supreme Tomato) 120
basil (*Barilla*) 70
basil (*Prego/Prego Extra Chunky* Zesty) 110
basil or mushroom and ripe olive (*Classico* Di Napoli/Di Sicilia) 50
cheese, three (*Prego*) 100
cheese, four (*Classico* Di Parma) 70
garden, combination (*Prego Extra Chunky*) 90
garlic or garlic and cheese (*Prego Extra Chunky* Supreme) 130

marinara (*Aunt Millie's*) 70
marinara (*Prego*) 110
marinara or mushroom and garlic (*Barilla*) 80
meat (*Prego*) 140
mushroom (*Prego*) 150
mushroom (*Prego Extra Chunky* Supreme) 130
mushroom with extra spice (*Prego Extra Chunky*) 120
mushroom and green pepper (*Prego Extra Chunky*) 120
mushroom and onion (*Prego Extra Chunky*) 110
mushroom, Parmesan (*Prego*) 120
mushroom and tomato (*Prego Extra Chunky*) 110
olive, green and black (*Barilla*) 100
onion and garlic or sweet pepper and spice (*Classico* Di Sorrento) 80
oregano, zesty (*Prego Extra Chunky*) 140
with Parmesan (*Prego*) 120
pepper, sweet and garlic (*Barilla*) 70
pepper, sweet and onion (*Classico* Di Salerno) 70
pepper, sweet and spicy (*Classico* Di Roma Arrabbiata) . 60
sausage, Italian and fennel (*Classico* D'Abruzzi) 90
spinach, Florentine, and cheese (*Classico* Di Firenze) 80
sun-dried tomato (*Classico* Di Capri) 80
with vegetables (*Prego Extra Chunky* Supreme) 90
zucchini and Parmesan (*Classico* Di Milano) 60

Pasta sauce, refrigerated, tomato (see also specific sauce listings):
marinara (*Contadina*), ½ cup 80
roasted garlic and artichoke (*Monterey Pasta Company*), ½ cup 70

Pastrami (see also "Turkey pastrami"), beef:
(*Healthy Deli*), 2 oz. 80
brisket or Romanian (*Boar's Head*), 2 oz. 90
round (*Boar's Head*), 2 oz. 70

Pastry filling (see also "Pie filling"), canned, 2 tbsp.:
almond (*Solo*) 120
apricot, Dutch apple, blueberry, cherry, pineapple, or raspberry (*Solo*) 80
date (*Solo*) 100
pecan (*Solo*) 130

Pastry filling ***(cont.)***
poppy seed or fancy nut (*Solo*) 140
prune plum or strawberry (*Solo*) 70
Pastry shell (see also "Pie crust"):
patty (*Pepperidge Farm*), 1 shell 230
sheet, puff (*Pepperidge Farm*), 1/6 sheet 200
tart (*Oronoque/Pet-Ritz*), 3" shell 140
Pâté (see also "Liverwurst"), canned:
chicken liver, 1 tbsp. 26
goose liver, smoked, 1 tbsp. 60
Pâté, vegetarian (*Bonavita* Swiss), 1 oz. 61
Peach, 1/2 cup, except as noted:
fresh, 2 1/2"-diam. peach or 1/2 cup slices 37
canned (*S&W* Natural/*S&W* Ready-Cut California/Tropical Sun) 80
canned, in heavy syrup, cling or freestone (*S&W*) 100
frozen, sliced, sweetened 118
sun-dried (*Del Monte*), 1/3 cup, 1.4 oz. 90
Peach drink (*Tree Top* Peach Quake), 8 fl. oz. 120
Peach dumpling, frozen (*Pepperidge Farm*), 1 piece . . . 300
Peach juice:
(*After the Fall* Georgia), 8 fl. oz. 100
blend (*Dole* Orchard), 8 fl. oz. 140
Peach nectar (*Libby's*), 8 fl. oz. 150
Peanut, shelled:
dry-roasted or honey-roasted (*Planters*), 1 oz. 160
honey-roasted (*Frito-Lay*), 1/4 cup 270
hot and spicy (*Planters Heat*), 1 oz. 160
oil-roasted (*Planters*), 2-oz. bag 340
oil-roasted, salted or cocktail (*Planters*), 1 oz. 170
Spanish (*Planters*), 1 oz. 170
Peanut butter, all varieties (*Skippy*), 2 tbsp. 190
Peanut sauce, Oriental:
(*House of Tsang Bangkok Padang*), 1 tbsp. 45
cooking (*Kylin Singapore Satay*), 1/4 cup 60
Pear, 1/2 cup, except as noted:
fresh, Bartlett, with peel, 1 medium, 2 1/2 per lb. 98
canned (*S&W* Ready-Cut California Sun) 80
canned, Bartlett, in juice (*S&W* Natural Style) 80

canned, Bartlett, in heavy syrup (*S&W*) 90
dried (*Sonoma*), 3–4 pieces, 1.4 oz. 120
Pear, Asian, whole, 1 medium, 2¼" × 2½" diam. 51
Pear juice:
(*After the Fall* Rouge River), 8 fl. oz. 100
(*R.W. Knudsen*), 8 fl. oz. 120
Pear nectar (*Libby's*), 8 fl. oz. 150
Peas, cream, canned (*Allens/East Texas Fair*), ½ cup . . 100
Peas, crowder, canned (*Allens/East Texas Fair/ Homefolks*), ½ cup 110
Peas, edible-podded:
fresh, raw, ½ cup 30
fresh, boiled, drained, ½ cup 34
fresh, sugar snap (*Frieda's*), 1 oz. 15
frozen, sugar snap (*Green Giant*), ¾ cup 35
Peas, field, canned:
fresh shell (*Sunshine*), ½ cup 120
dry, with bacon (*Trappey's*), ½ cup 90
Peas, green, sweet:
fresh, boiled, drained, ½ cup 67
canned (*S&W* Petit Pois/Sweet), ½ cup 70
canned (*Stokely/Stokely* No Salt), ½ cup 60
frozen (*Seabrook*), ⅔ cup 70
frozen, baby sweet or early June (*Green Giant LeSueur*), ⅔ cup 60
frozen, baby, early (*Green Giant Harvest Fresh/LeSueur*), ⅔ cup 70
frozen, in butter sauce (*Green Giant/LeSueur*), ¾ cup . . 100
Peas, green, combinations:
canned, with mushrooms and onions (*Green Giant LeSueur*), ½ cup 60
canned, with pearl onions (*S&W*), ½ cup 40
frozen, with mushrooms (*Green Giant LeSueur*), ¾ cup . 60
frozen, with pearl onions (*Green Giant*), ⅔ cup 60
Peas, lady, canned, with snaps (*Sunshine/East Texas Fair*), ½ cup 100
Peas, pepper, canned (*Allens/East Texas Fair/ Homefolks*), ½ cup 120
Peas, purple hull, canned (*East Texas*), ½ cup 120

Peas, split, see "Split peas"
Peas, sprouted, mature seeds, raw, 1/2 cup 77
Peas, white acre, canned (*East Texas Fair*), 1/2 cup 100
Peas and carrots, canned:
(*Stokely*), 1/2 cup 60
(*Stokely* No Salt/Sugar), 1/2 cup 50
Pecan, shelled:
chips, halves or pieces (*Planters*), 2-oz. pkg. 390
dry-roasted, 1 oz. 187
honey-roasted (*Planters*), 1 oz. 180
oil-roasted, 1 oz. 195
Penne dishes, mix, dry:
Alfredo (*Knorr*), 3/4 cup 280
herb and garlic (*Golden Saute*), 1/2 pkg. 230
with sun-dried tomato Parmesan (*Knorr*), 1/2 cup 270
Pepper, banana, hot or mild (*Vlasic*), 1 oz. 5
Pepper, cherry:
hot or mild (*Vlasic*), 1 oz. 10
marinated, drained (*Progresso*), 2 tbsp. 30
Pepper, chili:
raw, green or red, seeded, chopped, 1/2 cup 30
in jars, green, whole or diced (*Chi-Chi's*), 3/4 chili or
2 tbsp. 10
in jars, yellow, hot (*Del Monte*), 4 pieces, 1 oz. 10
Pepper, chili, relish, pickle (*Patak's*), 1 tbsp. 45
Pepper, chilpotle, spice sauce (*Del Monte*), 2 tbsp. 20
Pepper, jalapeño:
whole (*Del Monte*), .7-oz. piece 3
diced, marinated, or pickled (*La Victoria*), 1.1 oz. 10
Pepper, sweet:
fresh, green or red, raw, 1 medium, 3 3/4" × 3" diam. 20
fresh, yellow, raw, 1 large, 5" × 3" diam. 50
in jars, rings (*Vlasic*), 1 oz. 25
in jars, fire-roasted, with garlic, in oil (*Paesana*), 2 tbsp. . 20
in jars, roasted (*Progresso*), 1/2 piece 10
Pepper salad (*B&G*), 1 oz. 10
Pepper sauce:
(*Pickapeppa*), 1 tbsp. 18
all varieties (*Tabasco*), 1 tsp. 0

Pepperoncini:
(*Zorba*), 5 pieces, 1.1 oz. 15
salad (*Vlasic*), 1 oz. 5
Pepperoni (*Hormel/Leoni/Rosa Grande*), 1 oz. 140
Perch, meat only, baked, broiled, or microwaved, 4 oz. 133
Perch, ocean, see "Ocean perch"
Persimmon, fresh:
fuyu (*Frieda's*), 1 oz. 22
hachiya, trimmed (*Frieda's*), 1 oz. 36
Persimmon, dried, Japanese, 1 oz. 78
Pesto sauce:
in jars, tomato and (*Classico* Di Genoa), 1/2 cup 90
refrigerated, basil (*Contadina*), 1/4 cup 310
refrigerated, sun-dried tomato (*Contadina*), 1/4 cup 250
Pesto sauce mix:
red bell pepper (*Knorr*), 1/3 pkg. 30
tomato, sun-dried (*Knorr*), 1/3 pkg. 45
Pheasant, raw, meat with skin, 4 oz. 205
Picante sauce (see also "Salsa"), 2 tbsp.:
(*Pace*) 10
all varieties (*Hunt's* Homestyle) 10
black bean, black-eyed pea, or garlic with corn and honey (*Arthur's*) 15
hot, mild, or mesquite (*Arthur's*) 10
Pickle, cucumber (see also specific listings):
bread and butter, midgets (*Vlasic* Milwaukee), 1 oz. 40
bread and butter, sandwich stackers (*Vlasic*), 1 oz. 30
dill, all varieties (*Vlasic/Vlasic* Milwaukee), 1 oz. 5
kosher, regular or sour (*Hebrew National/Rosoff/Shorr's*), 1 oz. 4
sour (*Claussen* New York Deli), 1/2 pickle, 1 oz. 5
sweet, all varieties (*Vlasic*), 1 oz. 40
Pickle and pepper loaf (*Boar's Head*), 2 oz. 150
Pickle and pimiento loaf (*Oscar Mayer*), 1-oz. slice 70
Pickle relish, cucumber (see also specific relish listings):
hamburger (*Del Monte*), 1 tbsp. 20
hot dog (*Del Monte*), 1 tbsp. 15
piccalilli, tomato (*Pickle Eater's*), 1 tbsp. 10

Pickle relish *(cont.)*
sweet pickle, regular or curry flavor (*Vlasic*), 1 tbsp. 15
Pie, frozen:
apple (*Banquet*), 1/5 pie 300
apple, Dutch (*Mrs. Smith's* 8"), 1/6 pie 320
apple-cranberry (*Mrs. Smith's* 8"), 1/6 pie 280
berry, blackberry, or raspberry (*Mrs. Smith's* 8"), 1/6 pie 280
blueberry (*Mrs. Smith's* 8"), 1/6 pie 260
cherry (*Banquet*), 1/5 pie 290
cherry (*Mrs. Smith's* 8"), 1/6 pie 270
cream, banana or coconut (*Banquet*), 1/3 pie 350
cream, banana, coconut, or lemon (*Pet-Ritz*), 1/4 pie . . . 270
cream, chocolate or lemon (*Banquet*), 1/3 pie 360
cream, chocolate (*Sara Lee* Homestyle), 1/5 pie 500
lemon meringue (*Sara Lee* Homestyle), 1/6 pie 350
mincemeat (*Banquet*), 1/5 pie 310
peach (*Banquet*), 1/5 pie 260
pecan (*Mrs. Smith's* 8"), 1/6 pie 520
pumpkin (*Banquet*), 1/5 pie 250
pumpkin, hearty (*Mrs. Smith's* 8"), 1/5 pie 250
strawberry or strawberry-rhubarb (*Mrs. Smith's*8"),
1/5 pie 280
Pie, mix*, 1/6 pie:
chocolate silk (*Jell-O*) 310
coconut cream (*Jell-O*) 330
Pie, snack, 1 pie, except as noted:
apple (*Hostess*) 410
blackberry, blueberry, peach, or pineapple (*Hostess*) . . . 400
cherry (*Hostess*) 430
lemon (*Hostess*) 420
marshmallow, banana or chocolate (*Little Debbie*) 320
oatmeal creme (*Little Debbie*) 300
raisin creme (*Little Debbie*) 270
strawberry (*Hostess*) 390
Pie crust:
chocolate (*Ready Crust* 9"), 1/8 crust 110
cookie crumbs (*Oreo*), 2 tbsp. 80
graham (*Honey Maid*), 1/6 crust 140
graham crumbs (*Honey Maid*), 2 tbsp. 70

shortbread (*Ready Crust* 9″), 1/8 crust 100
vanilla cookie (*Nilla*), 1/6 crust 140
Pie crust, frozen or refrigerated, 1/8 crust:
(*Pet-Ritz* 9″) 80
deep dish, regular or vegetable shortening (*Pet-Ritz*) . . . 100
graham (*Pet Ritz*) 110
vegetable shortening (*Pet-Ritz*) 90
Pie crust mix (*Betty Crocker*), 1/8 of 9″ crust 110
Pie filling (see also "Pastry filling"), 1/3 cup, except as noted:
apple or apricot (*Lucky Leaf*) 90
blackberry or strawberry-rhubarb (*Lucky Leaf*) 90
blueberry (*Lucky Leaf/Lucky Leaf* Premium/*Musselman's*) 100
cherry (*Lucky Leaf/Lucky Leaf* Premium/*Musselman's*) . . 100
cherry, dark sweet (*Lucky Leaf/Musselman's*) 110
coconut or lemon creme (*Lucky Leaf/Musselman's* 22 oz.) 110
mincemeat (*Borden None Such*) 190
mincemeat (*Lucky Leaf*) 140
peach (*Lucky Leaf*) 80
pineapple or strawberry (*Lucky Leaf/Musselman's*) 100
pumpkin, mix (*Libby's*), 1/2 cup 100
raisin (*Lucky Leaf/Musselman's*) 100
Pierogies, frozen:
potato cheese (*Empire* Kosher), 4 oz. 214
potato onion (*Empire* Kosher), 4 oz. 165
potato onion (*Giorgio*), 3 pieces 230
Pigeon peas, fresh, boiled, drained, 1/2 cup 86
Pig's feet:
fresh, simmered, 4 oz. 220
pickled (*Hormel*), 2 oz. 80
Pike, meat only:
northern, baked, broiled, or microwaved, 4 oz. 128
walleye, baked, broiled, or microwaved, 4 oz. 135
Pimiento, drained, whole (*S&W*), 2 1/4 oz. 20
Piña colada mixer:
bottled (*Holland House*), 4.5 fl. oz. 180
canned (*Goya*), 1/3 cup 120
frozen* (*Bacardi*), 8 fl. oz. 190

Piña colada mixer *(cont.)*
mix (*Bar-Tenders*), 1.2-oz. pkt. 140
Pine nuts, dried:
pignolia (*Krinos*), .5 oz. 90
pinyon, 1 oz. 161
Pineapple, 1/2 cup, except as noted:
fresh, sliced (*Dole*), 2 slices 90
canned, in juice, all varieties, except sliced (*Del Monte*) . 70
canned, in juice, sliced (*Del Monte*), 2 slices 60
canned, in light syrup, all varieties, except sliced (*Dole*) . 80
canned, in light syrup, sliced (*Dole*), 4 oz., 3 1/2 slices 60
canned, in heavy syrup, all varieties (*Dole*), 1/2 cup or
2 slices 90
canned, in extra heavy syrup, crushed (*Dole*) 110
canned, in extra heavy syrup, cubes (*Dole*) 200
dried (*Sonoma*), 2 pieces, 1.4 oz. 140
frozen, sweetened, chunks 104
Pineapple drink, 8 fl. oz.:
(*Tropicana* Punch) 120
coconut (*Farmer's Market*) 120
grapefruit, pink (*Dole*) 130
Pineapple juice:
canned (*Dole*), 8 fl. oz. 120
chilled or frozen* (*Dole*), 8 fl. oz. 130
Pineapple juice blend, 8 fl. oz.:
coconut (*R.W. Knudsen*) 130
grapefruit, frozen* (*Dole*) 130
orange, orange-guava, or passion fruit–banana (*Dole*) . . 120
orange-banana, orange-berry, or orange-strawberry
(*Dole*) 130
Pink beans, canned, in tomato sauce (*Goya*), 1/2 cup . . . 100
Pinquito beans, canned (*S&W*), 1/2 cup 80
Pinto beans, canned:
(*Gebhardt*), 1/2 cup 90
(*Stokely*), 1/2 cup 110
with bacon (*Trappey's/Trappey's* Jalapinto), 1/2 cup 120
Pistachio nuts:
dried, in shell (*Dole*), 1 oz. 90
dried, shelled (*Dole*), 1 oz. 163

dry-roasted, shelled (*Planters*), 1 oz. 160
Pitanga, 1/2 cup 29
Pizza, frozen:
artichoke hearts (*Wolfgang Puck* 10″), 1/2 pie 340
Canadian bacon (*Tombstone* Original 12″), 1/4 pie 360
cheese (*Swanson Fun Feast* Meal), 1 pkg. 350
cheese (*Tombstone For One* 1/2 Less Fat), 1 pie 360
cheese, extra (*Marie Callender's*), 1/2 pie 410
cheese, extra (*Tombstone* Original 12″), 1/4 pie 370
cheese, extra (*Tombstone For One*), 1 pie 540
cheese, three, Italian style (*Tombstone* ThinCrust), 1/4 pie 380
cheese, four (*Tombstone Special Order* 12″), 1/5 pie 400
chicken and broccoli (*Marie Callender's*), 1/2 pie 350
deluxe (*Marie Callender's*), 1/2 pie 380
deluxe (*Tombstone* Original 12″), 1/4 pie 320
hamburger (*Tombstone* Original 12″), 1/5 pie 320
meat, four (*Tombstone Special Order* 12″), 1/6 pie 350
meat, combo, Italian style (*Tombstone* ThinCrust), 1/4 pie 410
meat, five, combo (*Marie Callender's*), 1/2 pie 330
Mexican style, supreme taco (*Tombstone* ThinCrust),
1/4 pie 380
pepperoni (*Marie Callender's*), 1/2 pie 440
pepperoni (*Tombstone* Original 12″), 1/5 pie 340
pepperoni (*Tombstone For One*), 1 pie 540
pepperoni (*Tombstone For One* 1/2 Less Fat), 1 pie 400
pepperoni (*Tombstone Special Order* 12″), 1/6 pie 360
pepperoni, double cheese (*Tombstone Double Top*),
1/6 pie 350
pepperoni, Italian style (*Tombstone* ThinCrust), 1/4 pie . . 420
sausage (*Tombstone* Original 12″), 1/5 pie 320
sausage, double cheese (*Tombstone Double Top*), 1/6 pie 350
sausage, Italian (*Tombstone For One*), 1 pie 560
sausage, Italian, Italian style (*Tombstone* ThinCrust),
1/4 pie 400
sausage, three (*Tombstone Special Order* 12″), 1/6 pie . . 340
sausage and mushroom (*Tombstone* Original 12″), 1/5 pie 320
sausage and pepperoni (*Marie Callender's*), 1/2 pie 430
sausage and pepperoni (*Tombstone For One*), 1 pie . . . 590
sausage, double cheese (*Tombstone Double Top*), 1/6 pie 360

Pizza *(cont.)*
supreme (*Tombstone* Original 12″), 1/5 pie 330
supreme (*Tombstone For One* 1/2 Less Fat), 1 pie 400
supreme, Italian style (*Tombstone* ThinCrust), 1/4 pie . . . 400
supreme (*Tombstone For One*), 1 pie 570
supreme, super (*Tombstone Special Order* 12″), 1/6 pie . . 350
vegetable (*Tombstone For One* 1/2 Less Fat), 1 pie 360
vegetable primavera (*Marie Callender's*), 1/2 pie 350
Pizza, French bread, frozen:
cheese (*Healthy Choice*), 1 piece 310
cheese (*Lean Cuisine*), 6 oz. 350
cheese (*Stouffer's*), 1/2 pkg. 350
cheese, double (*Stouffer's*), 1/2 pkg. 420
deluxe (*Lean Cuisine*), 6 1/8 oz. 330
deluxe (*Stouffer's*), 1/2 pkg. 440
pepperoni (*Healthy Choice*), 1 piece 360
pepperoni (*Lean Cuisine*), 5 1/4 oz. 330
pepperoni or sausage (*Stouffer's*), 1/2 pkg. 420
pepperoni and mushroom (*Stouffer's*), 1/2 pkg. 430
sausage (*Healthy Choice*), 1 piece 330
sausage and pepperoni or white pizza (*Stouffer's*),
1/2 pkg. 490
supreme (*Healthy Choice*), 1 piece 340
vegetable, deluxe (*Stouffer's*), 1/2 pkg. 400
Pizza, Italian bread, 1 piece:
cheese, four (*Celeste*) 300
chicken, zesty (*Celeste*) 260
deluxe (*Celeste*) 290
pepperoni (*Celeste*) 320
Pizza crust, refrigerated (*Pillsbury*), 1/4 crust 180
Pizza Hut:
Bigfoot, cheese, 1 slice 186
Bigfoot, pepperoni, 1 slice 205
Bigfoot, pepperoni, mushroom, and sausage, 1 slice . . . 214
breadsticks, 5 pieces 750
hand-tossed, 1 slice of medium pie:
cheese 235
beef 260
ham 213

Meat Lovers 314
pepperoni 238
Pepperoni Lovers 306
pork topping 268
sausage, Italian 267
supreme 284
supreme, super 296
Veggie Lovers 216
pan pizza, 1 slice of medium pie:
cheese 261
beef 286
ham 239
Meat Lovers 340
pepperoni 265
Pepperoni Lovers 332
pork topping 294
sausage, Italian 293
supreme 311
supreme, super 323
Veggie Lovers 243
Personal Pan Pizza, pepperoni, 1 pie 637
Personal Pan Pizza, supreme, 1 pie 722
Thin 'N Crispy, 1 slice of medium pie:
cheese 205
beef 229
ham 184
Meat Lovers 288
pepperoni 215
Pepperoni Lovers 289
pork topping 237
sausage, Italian 236
supreme 257
supreme, super 270
Veggie Lovers 186
Pizza nuggets, frozen (*Hormel Quick Meal*), 5 pieces,
2.8 oz. 210
Pizza pocket, frozen, 1 piece:
(*Amy's*) 290
deluxe (*Lean Pockets*) 270

Pizza pocket *(cont.)*
pepperoni (*Croissant Pockets*) 350
pepperoni (*Hot Pockets*) 350
pepperoni and sausage or sausage (*Hot Pockets*) 340
vegetable (*Ken & Robert's Veggie Pockets*) 270
vegetable, pepperoni style (*Amy's*) 220
Pizza sauce, 1/4 cup:
(*Contadina*) 25
(*Contadina Pizza Squeeze*) 35
(*Prince* Traditional) 20
with Italian cheese or pepperoni (*Contadina*) 30
Plantain:
raw (*Frieda's*), 1 oz. 34
cooked, sliced, 1/2 cup 89
fried (*Goya* Tostone), 3 pieces 170
Plum:
fresh, Japanese or hybrid, 1 medium, 2 1/8" diam. 36
canned in juice, 3 plums and 2 tbsp. liquid 55
canned in light syrup, 3 plums and 2 3/4 tbsp. liquid 83
canned in heavy syrup, whole (*S&W*), 1/2 cup 130
Plum sauce:
(*Ka-Me*), 2 tbsp. 80
(*La Choy*), 1 tbsp. 25
Poke greens, canned (*Allens*), 1/2 cup 35
Polenta, prepared:
(*Frieda's*), 4 oz. 100
(*San Gennaro's*), 3.5 oz. 70
Polenta mix* (*Fantastica*), 1 cup 260
Polish sausage (see also "Kielbasa"):
beef (*Hebrew National*), 3-oz. link 240
beef (*Hebrew National* Quarter Pound), 4-oz. link 330
skinless (*John Morrell*), 2 oz. 180
Pollock, meat only, 4 oz.:
Atlantic, baked, broiled, or microwaved 134
walleye, baked, broiled, or microwaved 128
Pomegranate, 1 medium, 9.7 oz. 104
Pomegranate juice (*R.W. Knudsen*), 8 fl. oz. 150
Pompano, Florida, meat only, baked, broiled, or
microwaved, 4 oz. 239

Popcorn, unpopped, 2 tbsp.:
regular or hot air (*Orville Redenbacher* Original or White) . 90
microwave (*Orville Redenbacher*) 120
microwave, butter flavor (*Orville Redenbacher*) 170
microwave, caramel or herb and garlic (*Orville Redenbacher*) 180
microwave, cheddar (*Orville Redenbacher*) 140
microwave, natural flavor (*Orville Redenbacher*) 160
Popcorn, popped:
(*Barrel O'Fun* Canola), 3 cups 145
butter flavor (*Smartfood*), 3 cups 150
caramel (*Barrel O'Fun* Fat Free), 3/4 cup 120
caramel, with peanuts (*Barrel O'Fun*), 2/3 cup 130
caramel, with peanuts (*Cracker Jack*), 2/3 cup 120
cheddar, white (*Barrel O'Fun*), 3 cups 185
cheddar, white (*Smartfood*), 2 cups 190
cheese (*Barrel O'Fun* Cheesecorn), 2 1/2 cups 135
microwave (*Jolly Time* Natural), 4 cups 160
microwave, air-popped, white or yellow (*Jolly Time*), 5 cups 100
microwave, butter flavor (*Jolly Time*), 4 cups 140
microwave, nacho (*Pop Secret*), 1 cup 30
toffee crunch (*Smartfood*), 3/4 cup 130
Popcorn bar, caramel or chocolate (*Pop Secret*), 1 bar . 70
Popcorn cakes:
butter (*Orville Redenbacher*), 3 cakes 115
caramel (*Orville Redenbacher*), 2 cakes 80
cheddar, white (*Orville Redenbacher*), 3 cakes 110
Pork, fresh (see also "Ham"), meat only, 4 oz., except as noted:
loin, center, broiled, lean with fat 358
loin, center, broiled, lean only 262
loin, center, roasted, lean with fat 346
loin, center, roasted, lean only 272
loin, center, rib, broiled, lean with fat 389
loin, center, rib, broiled, lean only 293
loin, center, rib, roasted, lean with fat 361
loin, center, rib, roasted, lean only 278
loin, top, broiled, lean with fat 408

Pork *(cont.)*
loin, top, broiled, lean only 293
loin, top, roasted, lean only 278
shoulder, arm (picnic), roasted, lean with fat 375
shoulder, arm (picnic), roasted, lean only 259
shoulder, Boston blade, braised, lean with fat 421
shoulder, Boston blade, braised, lean only 333
shoulder, Boston blade, roasted, lean only 290
sirloin, broiled, lean with fat 375
sirloin, broiled, lean only 276
sirloin, roasted, lean with fat 330
sirloin, roasted, lean only 268
spareribs, lean with fat, braised, 6.3 oz. (1 lb. raw with bone) 703
tenderloin, lean only, roasted 188
Pork, cured (see also "Ham"), 4 oz.:
arm (picnic), roasted, lean with fat 318
arm (picnic), roasted, lean only 193
blade roll, lean with fat, roasted 325
Pork, pickled (see also "Pig's feet"):
hocks (*Hormel*), 2 oz. 110
tidbits (*Hormel*), 2 oz. 100
Pork, refrigerated:
loin, center cut (*John Morrell Table Trim*), 4 oz. 190
smoked shoulder butt (*Oscar Mayer Sweet Morsel*), 3 oz. 180
tenderloin (*John Morrell Table Trim*), 4 oz. 120
Pork batter, frying (*House of Tsang*), 4 tbsp. 140
Pork dinner, rib-shape, frozen (*Swanson Hungry Man*), 1 pkg. 770
Pork entree, canned, chow mein (*La Choy* Bi-Pack), 1 cup 80
Pork entree, frozen:
cutlet (*Banquet*), 10.25 oz. 410
ribs, barbecue sauce (*Swanson Fun Feast*), 1 pkg. 450
rib-shape patty, barbecue (*Swanson*), 1 pkg. 460
sweet and sour (*Chun King*), 13 oz. 450
Pork gravy (*Franco-American*), 1/4 cup 45
Pork gravy mix (*Durkee/French's*), 1/4 cup* 10

Pork lunch meat:
(*Hormel Deli Pork Roast*), 2 oz. 70
seasoned (*Boar's Head*), 2 oz. 80
Pork rind snack, .5 oz.:
(*Old Dutch Bac'n Puffs*) 80
(*Baken-ets/Baken-ets* Cracklins) 80
hot and spicy (*Baken-ets*) 70
Pork sandwich, frozen, barbecued (*Hormel Quick Meal*), 1 piece 350
Pork seasoning mix:
(*Shake'n Bake* Original Recipe), 1/8 pkg. 40
barbecue glaze (*Shake'n Bake*), 1/8 pkg. 35
extra crispy (*Oven Fry*), 1/8 pkg. 60
hot and spicy (*Shake'n Bake*), 1/8 pkg. 45
Pot roast, see "Beef dinner" and "Beef entree"
Pot roast seasoning mix:
(*Lawry's*), 1 tsp. 5
sauerbraten (*Knorr* Recipe), 1/6 pkg. 35
Potato (see also "Sweet potato"):
baked in skin, 1 medium, 4 3/4" × 2 1/3" diam. 220
baked without skin, 1/2 cup 57
boiled in skin, baby (*Frieda's*), 4 oz. 86
boiled in skin, peeled, 1/2 cup 68
boiled without skin, 1/2 cup 67
microwaved in skin, 1 medium, 4 3/4" × 2 1/3" diam. 212
microwaved in skin, peeled, 1/2 cup 78
mashed, with whole milk, 1/2 cup 81
Potato, canned (see also "Potato dishes, canned"):
whole (*Stokely/Stokely* No Salt), 5.5 oz. 80
whole, new (*S&W*), 1/2 cup 60
mashed (*Idahoan* Real), 1/3 cup 80
Potato, frozen (see also "Potato dishes, frozen"):
(*Ore-Ida* Deep Fries/Deep Fries Crinkle Cuts), 3 oz. 160
(*Ore-Ida* Shoestring/*Ore-Ida Homestyle Wedges With Skin*), 3 oz. 150
(*Ore-Ida* Steak Fries), 3 oz. 110
(*Ore-Ida Crispers!*), 3 oz. 220
(*Ore-Ida Crispy Crowns!*), 3 oz. 190
(*Ore-Ida Crispy Crunchies!/Ore-Ida Zesties*), 3 oz. 160

Potato, frozen ***(cont.)***
(*Ore-Ida Fast Fries/Golden Twirls/Waffle Fries*), 3 oz. . . . 150
(*Ore-Ida Golden Crinkles*), 3 oz. 140
(*Ore-Ida Golden Fries*), 3 oz. 120
(*Ore-Ida Golden Pixie Crinkles*), 3 oz. 130
(*Ore-Ida Snackin' Fries*), 5-oz. pkg. 340
(*Ore-Ida Texas Crispers!*), 3 oz. 170
cottage fries (*Ore-Ida*), 3 oz. 130
country fries (*Ore-Ida*), 3 oz. 120
country fries, ranch flavor (*Ore-Ida Fast Fries*), 3 oz. . . . 150
country fries, zesty (*Ore-Ida Snackin' Fries*), 5-oz. pkg. . . 340
hash brown (*Ore-Ida Golden Patties*), 1 patty 160
hash brown (*Ore-Ida* Microwave), 4-oz. pkg. 220
hash brown, with cheddar (*Ore-Ida Cheddar Browns*),
  1 patty 80
hash brown, country style (*Ore-Ida*), 1 cup 60
hash brown, shredded (*Ore-Ida*), 1 patty 70
hash brown, Southern style (*Ore-Ida*), 3/4 cup 80
hash brown, toaster (*Ore-Ida*), 2 patties 190
mashed (*Ore-Ida*), 2/3 cup 90
O'Brien (*Ore-Ida*), 3/4 cup 60
puffs (*Hot Tots/Tater Tots*), 3 oz. 160
puffs (*Tater Tots* Microwave), 4-oz. pkg. 180
Potato, mix (see also "Potato pancake mix"), dry:
(*Betty Crocker Potato Buds*), 1/3 cup 80
au gratin (*Idahoan*), 1/3 cup 110
cheddar and sour cream (*Betty Crocker*), 2/3 cup 120
mashed (*Idahoan* Flakes), 1/3 cup 80
mashed (*Pillsbury* Idaho), 2 tbsp. 90
scalloped (*Betty Crocker*), 2/3 cup 100
scalloped (*Idahoan*), 1/3 cup 110
scalloped, cheesy (*Betty Crocker*), 1/2 cup 90
vegetable and herb (*Good Harvest*), 1/3 cup 110
Western (*Idahoan*), 1/4 cup 100
Potato chips (see also "Potato sticks"), 1 oz., except as
  noted:
(*Lay's*) 150
(*Lay's* Wavy) 160
(*Munchos*) 150

(*Ruffles*) 150
(*Ruffles* Reduced Fat) 140
all flavors, except barbecue and onion and garlic (*Barrel O'Fun*) 150
all flavors (*Lay's* Baked) 110
barbecue (*Barrel O'Fun*) 145
barbecue, mesquite (*Ruffles KC Masterpiece*) 150
cheddar and sour cream (*Ruffles*) 160
cheddar and sour cream (*Wise*) 150
Dijon, golden (*Ruffles*) 150
onion, French (*Ruffles*) 150
onion and garlic (*Barrel O'Fun*) 140
ranch (*Ruffles*) 150
sour cream and onion (*Ruffles* Reduced Fat) 130
Potato dishes, canned, 7.5 oz.:
au gratin, and bacon (*Hormel*) 250
scalloped, and ham (*Hormel*) 260
sliced, and beef (*Dinty Moore*) 230
Potato dishes, frozen:
au gratin (*Stouffer's* Side Dish), 4.6 oz. 130
baked, broccoli-cheddar (*Lean Cuisine Lunch Express* Entree), 10 oz. 220
baked, broccoli-cheese (*Ore-Ida* Twice Baked), 6 oz. . . . 150
baked, broccoli-cheese (*Weight Watchers* Entree), 10 oz. 250
baked, butter flavor (*Ore-Ida* Twice Baked), 5 oz. 200
baked, cheddar (*Ore-Ida* Twice Baked), 5 oz. 190
baked, sour cream–chives (*Ore-Ida* Twice Baked), 5 oz. 190
cheddar (*Lean Cuisine* Entree Deluxe), 10⅜ oz. 230
cheddar pocket (*Ken & Robert's Veggie Pockets*), 1 piece 260
scalloped (*Stouffer's* Side Dish), 4.6 oz. 140
scalloped, and ham (*Swanson* Entree), 1 pkg. 290
Potato flour, 1 cup 628
Potato pancake, frozen:
(*Empire* Kosher), 2-oz. cake 80
mini (*Empire* Kosher), 2 cakes, 2 oz. 90
Potato pancake mix (*Knorr*), 2 tbsp. 80
Potato seasoning:
cheddar, savory (*Lipton Recipe Secrets*), 1 tbsp. 60

Potato seasoning *(cont.)*
garlic herb (*Lipton Recipe Secrets*), 1 tbsp. 50
onion, California (*Lipton Recipe Secrets*), 1 tbsp. 60
Potato seasoning mix:
(*Potato Shakers*), 3 tsp. 30
cheddar, crispy (*Shake 'n Bake Perfect Potatoes*), 1/6 pkg. . 30
herb garlic (*Shake 'n Bake Perfect Potatoes*), 1/6 pkg. 20
Potato sticks:
(*Butterfield*), 2/3 cup 150
(*Pik-Nik* Fabulous Fries), 2/3 cup, 1 oz. 150
hot (*Chester's* Fries Flamin'), 1 oz. 140
ketchup (*Pik-Nik* Ketchup 'n Fries), 2/3 cup, 1.1 oz. 160
shoestring (*Pik-Nik*), 2/3 cup, 1 oz. 160
shoestring, BBQ (*Pik-Nik*), 2/3 cup, 1.2 oz. 180
shoestring, sour cream and cheddar (*Pik-Nik*), 2/3 cup,
1.2 oz. 180
Pout, ocean, meat only, baked, broiled, or microwaved,
4 oz. 116
Preserves, see "Jam and preserves"
Pretzel (see also "Crackers"), 1 oz., except as noted:
(*Barrel O'Fun* Fat Free Minis) 105
(*Little Debbie*), 1.2 oz. 140
(*Pepperidge Farm Goldfish*), 45 pieces, 1.1 oz. 120
(*Mister Salty* Mini) 110
all flavors (*Combos*) 130
bagel shaped (*Manischewitz*), 4 pieces, 1 oz. 110
Bavarian (*Rold Gold*) 110
chips (*Mister Salty*) 110
Dutch (*Mister Salty*), 2 pieces, 1.1 oz. 120
soft (*Superpretzel/Superpretzel* Added Salt), 2.3-oz. piece 170
soft, bites (*Superpretzel/Superpretzel* Added Salt),
4 pieces, 1.5 oz. 110
soft, cheese-filled (*Superpretzel Softstix*), 2 pieces,
1.8 oz. 140
soft, cinnamon raisin (*Superpretzel*), 2 pieces, 2 oz. . . . 190
sticks or twists (*Mister Salty* Fat Free) 110
twists (*Planters*) 100
Prickly pear, 1 medium, 4.8 oz. 42
Prosciutto (*Primissimo*), 2 oz. 210

Prune:
canned, in heavy syrup, 5 medium and 2 tbsp. liquid 90
canned, in heavy syrup, (*Sonoma*), 3–4 pieces, 1.4 oz. . . 110
canned, in heavy syrup, stewed (*S&W*), 8 pieces, 4.9 oz. 210
dehydrated, uncooked, ½ cup 224
dried (*Del Monte*), 1.4 oz., ¼ cup 120
dried (*Dole*), 2 oz. 140
dried, pitted (*Sonoma*), ¼ cup 120
dried, stewed, with pits, unsweetened, ½ cup 113
Prune juice, 8 fl. oz.:
(*Lucky Leaf/Musselman's*) 160
(*R.W. Knudsen* Organic) 170
(*S&W*) 180
Pudding, ready-to-serve, 4 oz.:
banana (*Hunt's Snack Pack*) 160
banana (*Jell-O* Snack) 170
banana, nondairy (*Imagine*) 150
butterscotch (*Hunt's Snack Pack*) 150
butterscotch, nondairy (*Imagine*) 150
butterscotch or vanilla (*Swiss Miss*) 160
chocolate (*Hunt's Snack Pack* Fat Free) 100
chocolate (*Swiss Miss*) 170
chocolate, nondairy (*Imagine*) 170
chocolate or chocolate fudge (*Hunt's Snack Pack*) 170
chocolate or chocolate fudge (*Swiss Miss* Fat Free) 100
chocolate or vanilla (*Jell-O* Snack) 160
chocolate fudge (*Swiss Miss*) 175
chocolate fudge, parfait (*Swiss Miss*) 160
chocolate marshmallow (*Hunt's Snack Pack*) 155
chocolate vanilla parfait (*Swiss Miss*) 160
chocolate swirl, caramel (*Hunt's Snack Pack*) 170
chocolate swirl, caramel (*Swiss Miss*) 170
chocolate swirl, caramel or vanilla (*Jell-O* Snack) 160
chocolate swirl, caramel or vanilla (*Jell-O Free* Snack) . . 100
chocolate swirl, milk (*Hunt's Snack Pack*) 160
chocolate swirl, vanilla (*Swiss Miss*) 170
lemon or vanilla (*Hunt's Snack Pack*) 160
lemon, nondairy (*Imagine*) 150
S'mores swirl or tapioca (*Hunt's Snack Pack*) 150

Pudding *(cont.)*
tapioca (*Hunt's Snack Pack* Fat Free) 95
tapioca (*Jell-O* Snack) 140
tapioca (*Swiss Miss*) 140
tapioca (*Swiss Miss* Fat Free) 100
vanilla (*Hunt's Snack Pack* Fat Free) 95
vanilla (*Jell-O Free* Snack) 100
vanilla (*Swiss Miss* Fat Free) 100
vanilla chocolate, parfait (*Swiss Miss*) 160
vanilla chocolate, parfait (*Swiss Miss* Fat Free) 100
vanilla chocolate, swirl (*Jell-O* Snack) 170
vanilla chocolate, swirl (*Jell-O Free* Snack) 100
Pudding mix, ½ cup*, except as noted:
banana or butterscotch (*Jell-O* Sugar/Fat Free) 70
banana cream or butterscotch (*Jell-O* Instant) 150
banana cream or lemon (*Jell-O*) 140
butter pecan (*Jell-O* Instant) 160
butterscotch (*Jell-O*) 160
chocolate, all flavors (*Jell-O*) 150
chocolate, all flavors (*Jell-O* Instant) 160
chocolate or chocolate fudge (*Jell-O* Sugar/Fat Free) 80
chocolate mousse, dark or milk (*Alsa*), dry, 2 tbsp. 80
chocolate mousse, white (*Alsa*), dry, 2 tbsp. 70
coconut cream (*Jell-O*) 150
coconut cream or vanilla (*Jell-O* Instant) 160
custard or tapioca (*Jello-O Americana*) 140
flan (*Alsa* Creme Caramel), 1⅓ tbsp. mix and 1 tbsp.
caramel 110
flan (*Jell-O*) 140
lemon (*Jell-O* Instant) 150
pistachio (*Jell-O* Instant) 160
pistachio or vanilla (*Jell-O* Sugar/Fat Free) 70
rice, see "Rice pudding mix"
vanilla (*Jell-O*) 140
vanilla (*Jell-O* Sugar Free) 80
vanilla, French (*Jell-O* Instant) 150
Puff pastry, see "Pastry shell"
Pummelo:
1 medium, 5½" diam. 228

(*Frieda's*), 3.5 oz. 38
Pumpkin:
fresh, boiled, drained, mashed, ½ cup 24
canned (*Libby's*), ½ cup 60
canned (*Stokely*), ½ cup 50
Pumpkin butter (*Smucker's*), 1 tbsp. 45
Pumpkin flower, boiled, drained, ½ cup 10
Pumpkin leaf, boiled, drained, ½ cup 7
Pumpkin pie spice, 1 tsp. 6
Pumpkin seeds:
roasted, in shell, 1 oz. or 85 seeds 127
roasted, in shell, 1 cup 285
roasted, shelled, 1 oz. 148
dried, shelled, 1 oz. or 142 kernels 154
tamari-roasted, spicy (*Eden*), 1 oz. 170
Punch, see "Fruit drink blends" and specific fruit listings
Purslane:
raw, ½ cup 4
boiled, drained, ½ cup 10
Quail, raw:
meat only, 1 quail, 3.2 oz. (4.3 oz. with bone and skin) 123
breast meat only, 1 breast, 2 oz. 69
Quince:
1 medium, 5.3 oz. 53
pineapple, peeled, seeded (*Frieda's*), 3.5 oz. 57
Quinoa:
(*Eden*), ¼ cup 170
black and white (*Frieda's*), 2 oz. dry or ½ cup cooked . . 218

R

FOOD AND MEASURE	CALORIES
Rabbit, domesticated, meat only, roasted, 4 oz.	223
Radicchio, fresh, shredded, ½ cup	5
Radish:	
10 medium, ¾"–1" diam.	7
Oriental, boiled, drained, sliced, ½ cup	13
white icicle, sliced, ½ cup	7
Radish sprouts (*Jonathan's*), 1 cup	57
Rainbow baking morsels (*Nestlé*), 1 tbsp.	70
Raisin, ½ cup, except as noted:	
monukka or Thompson (*Sonoma*), ¼ cup	130
seedless or golden seedless (*Dole*), ½ cup	250
Raisin sauce (*Reese*), ¼ cup	150
Ranch dip, 2 tbsp.:	
(*Heluva* Good Classic)	60
(*Nalley's*)	110
(*Ruffles*)	70
(*Ruffles* Low Fat)	40
bacon (*Marie's*)	150
peppercorn (*Marie's* Fat Free)	35
Ranch dip mix, cracked pepper (*Knorr*), ½ tsp.	5
Raspberry, red:	
fresh, ½ cup	31
frozen, sweetened, ½ cup	129
Raspberry drink, 8 fl. oz., except as noted:	
(*Farmer's Market*)	120
hibiscus (*R.W. Knudsen*)	90
lemon splash (*Dole*), 16 fl. oz.	250
Raspberry juice, 8 fl. oz.:	
(*Heinke's* Mountain)	120
blend (*Dole* Country)	140
cranberry (*Apple & Eve*)	120
peach (*R.W. Knudsen*)	120
Raspberry nectar (*R.W. Knudsen*), 8 fl. oz.	120

Ravioli, canned, 1 cup, except as noted:
with meat (*Chef Boyardee*) 230
cheese, tomato sauce (*Chef Boyardee*) 210
cheese, with meat (*Chef Boyardee* Bowl), 7.5 oz. 190
Ravioli, frozen or refrigerated:
(*Monterey Pasta Company* Mediterranean), 3 oz. 250
cheddar roasted garlic, garlic basil cheese, gorgonzola roasted walnut, or smoked Monterey Jack (*Monterey Pasta Company*), 3 oz. 240
cheese, four (*Contadina*), 1 cup 280
crab, snow (*Monterey Pasta Company*), 3 oz. 230
garden vegetable (*Contadina* Light), 1 cup 240
parsley (*Putney*), 1 cup 250
Ravioli entree, cheese, frozen:
(*Lean Cuisine*), 8½ oz. 240
(*Swanson Fun Feast* Roarin'), 1 pkg. 440
Florentine (*Smart Ones*), 8½ oz. 190
in marinara sauce (*Marie Callender's*), 8 oz. 370
parmigiana (*Healthy Choice*), 9 oz. 250
Red beans (see also "Kidney beans" and "Mexican beans"), canned:
(*Allens*), ½ cup 160
(*Stokely*), ½ cup 110
small (*Hunt's*), ½ cup 90
Refried beans, canned, ½ cup:
(*Chi-Chi's*) 130
(*Chi-Chi's* Fat Free/Vegetarian) 80
(*Rosarita*) 125
(*Rosarita* No Fat) 110
with bacon or with onion (*Rosarita*) 115
black beans (*Las Palmas/Old El Paso*) 120
black beans (*Rosarito* Low Fat) 105
with cheese, nacho (*Rosarita*) 135
with green chilies (*Rosarita*) 110
spicy or vegetarian (*Rosarita*) 120
vegetarian (*Gebhardt*) 120
vegetarian (*Old El Paso*) 100
Refried beans, mix, (*Fantastic* Instant), ½ cup* 160
Relish, see "Pickle relish" and specific listings

Remoulade sauce (*Zararain's*), ¼ cup 80
Rennet (*Junket*), 1 tablet 1
Rhubarb, fresh, diced, ½ cup 13
Rhubarb, frozen, cooked, sweetened, ½ cup 139
Rice (see also "Wild rice"), ¼ cup dry, except as noted:
Arborio (*Fantastic Foods*) 210
Arborio, brown or white (*Lundberg Nutra-Farmed*) 160
basmati, brown (*Fantastic Foods*) 170
basmati, white (*Casbah*) 158
basmati, white (*Fantastic Foods*) 180
blend (*Lundberg Country Wild/Lundberg Wild Blend*) . . . 150
blend (*Lundberg Jubilee/Lundberg Japonica*) 170
brown (*Carolina/Mahatma/River*) 150
brown, long grain (*S&W*) 150
brown, long grain (*Uncle Ben's* Whole Grain) 170
brown, long grain (*Uncle Ben's* Instant), ½ cup 190
glutinous or sweet, ½ cup cooked 117
jasmine (*Fantastic Foods*) 170
white, long grain (*Carolina/Mahatma*) 150
white, long grain, instant (*Minute/Minute* Premium), ½ cup 170
white, long grain, parboiled (*Uncle Ben's Converted*) . . . 170
Rice bran, crude, 1 cup 262
Rice cakes (see also "Popcorn cakes"), 1 cake, except as noted:
plain (*Mother's* Mini Unsalted), 7 cakes 60
all varieties, bars (*Health Valley* Crisp Fat Free) 110
all varieties except cheddar (*Quaker* Mini), 5 cakes 50
apple cinnamon, cheddar, or garden vegetable (*Crispy Cakes*) 35
apple cinnamon or cinnamon crunch (*Quaker*) 50
brown, toasted (*Crispy Cakes*) 30
cheddar, white or nacho corn (*Quaker*) 40
cheese, cheddar, white (*Quaker* Mini), 6 cakes 50
pizza or ranch (*Crispy Cakes*) 30
Rice dishes, canned:
Chinese fried (*La Choy*), 1 cup 240
Spanish (*Old El Paso*), 1 cup 130
Spanish (*Van Camp's*), 1 cup 180

Rice dishes, mix, dry, except as noted:
and beans, all varieties, except red, pilaf (*Near East*), 2 oz. 270
and beans, black (*Carolina/Mahatma*), 2 oz. 200
and beans, black or red (*Goya*), ¼ cup 160
and beans, black or spicy red (*Spice Islands* Quick Meal), 1 pkg. 180
and beans, Cajun (*Lipton* Rice & Sauce), ½ pkg. 260
and beans, pinto or red (*Carolina/Mahatma*), 2 oz. 190
and beans, red, pilaf (*Near East*), 2 oz. 220
beef (*Golden Saute*), ⅓ pkg. 230
beef, regular or with broccoli (*Lipton* Rice & Sauce), ½ pkg. 230
beef or chicken (*Uncle Ben's Country Inn*), 2 oz. 200
beef or chicken pilaf (*Near East*), 2 oz. 220
broccoli, Alfredo or cheddar (*Lipton* Rice & Sauce), ½ pkg. 250
broccoli, au gratin (*Uncle Ben's Country Inn*), 2 oz. 200
broccoli, cheese (*Mahatma*), 2 oz. 200
Cajun (*Lipton* Rice & Sauce), ½ pkg. 230
cheese (*Uncle Ben's Country Inn*), 2 oz. 210
chicken (*Golden Saute*), ⅓ pkg. 240
chicken (*Lipton* Rice & Sauce), ½ pkg. 240
chicken, creamy (*Lipton* Rice & Sauce), ½ pkg. 260
chicken pilaf (*Spice Islands* Quick Meal), 1 pkg. 180
chicken and broccoli (*Golden Saute*), ½ pkg. 260
chicken and broccoli (*Lipton* Rice & Sauce), ½ pkg. . . . 250
chicken and broccoli (*Rice-A-Roni*), 1 cup* 290
chicken with broccoli or vegetables (*Uncle Ben's Country Inn*), 2 oz. 200
chicken and wild rice (*Uncle Ben's Country Inn*), 2 oz. . . 190
chili (*Lundberg One Step* Entree), 2 oz. 180
curry or garlic basil (*Lundberg One Step* Entree), 2 oz. . . 160
curry pilaf (*Near East*), 2 oz. 220
fried (*Golden Saute*), ½ pkg. 240
fried (*Rice-A-Roni*), 1 cup* 320
gumbo (*Mahatma*), 2 oz. 160
herb and butter (*Lipton* Rice & Sauce), ½ pkg. 240
herb and butter or savory herb (*Golden Saute*), ⅓ pkg. 240

Rice dishes, mix *(cont.)*

jambalaya or long grain and wild (*Mahatma*), 2 oz. 190
long grain and wild (*Lipton* Rice & Sauce), ½ pkg. 250
long grain and wild, herb, all varieties (*Uncle Ben's*), 2 oz. 200
long grain and wild, pilaf (*Near East*), 2 oz. 220
medley (*Lipton* Rice & Sauce), ½ pkg. 240
Mexican or primavera (*Goya*), ¼ cup 160
mushroom (*Lipton* Rice & Sauce), ½ pkg. 220
onion mushroom (*Golden Saute*), ⅓ pkg. 240
Oriental (*Golden Saute*), ⅓ pkg. 240
Oriental (*Lipton* Rice & Sauce), ½ pkg. 240
Oriental, and vegetables (*Spice Islands* Quick Meal), 1 pkg. 180
pilaf (*Mahatma*), 2 oz. 190
pilaf (*Uncle Ben's Country Inn*), 2 oz. 200
pilaf, almond, toasted (*Near East*), 2 oz. 230
pilaf, brown rice or white (*Near East*), 2 oz. 220
pilaf or chicken risotto (*Lipton* Rice & Sauce), ½ pkg. . . 230
risotto (*Rice-A-Roni*), 1 cup* 310
risotto, all varieties (*Lundberg*), ¼ cup 140
risotto, broccoli au gratin (*Knorr*), ⅓ cup 260
risotto, Milanese (*Knorr*), ⅓ cup 280
risotto, mushroom (*Knorr*), ⅓ cup 300
risotto, onion herb (*Knorr*), ⅓ cup 310
risotto, primavera (*Knorr*), ⅓ cup 290
Spanish (*Golden Saute*), ½ pkg. 250
Spanish (*Lipton* Rice & Sauce), ½ pkg. 240
Spanish (*Mahatma*), 2 oz. 180
Spanish (*Uncle Ben's Country Inn*), 2 oz. 200
Spanish, pilaf (*Near East*), 2 oz. 230
vegetable, country (*Spice Islands* Quick Meal), 1 pkg. . . 180
wild rice and vegetables (*Spice Islands* Quick Meal), 1 pkg. 170
yellow (*Goya*), ¼ cup 170
yellow, saffron (*Carolina/Mahatma*), 2 oz. 190

Rice entree, frozen:

and broccoli (*Green Giant*), 10 oz. 320
and chicken, stir-fry (*Lean Cuisine*), 9 oz. 280

fried, with chicken (*Chun King*), 8 oz. 270
fried, with pork (*Chun King*), 8 oz. 290
Mexican, with chicken (*Lean Cuisine*), 9 oz. 270
pilaf, and vegetables (*Green Giant*), 10 oz. 230
and vegetables (*Green Giant* Medley), 10 oz. 240
and vegetables, Oriental (*Green Giant* International), 8 oz. 180
white and wild, and vegetables (*Green Giant*), 10 oz. . . . 250

Rice flour:
brown (*Arrowhead Mills*), 1/4 cup 120
white (*Arrowhead Mills*), 1/4 cup 160

Rice pudding mix:
(*Goya*), 1/2 cup* 90
(*Jell-O Americana*), 1/2 cup* 160
cinnamon and raisin (*Uncle Ben's*), 1.5 oz. dry 160

Rigatoni, canned, Italian garden sauce (*Hunt's* Homestyle), 1 cup 165

Rigatoni entree, frozen:
(*Lean Cuisine*), 9 oz. 180
parmigiana (*Marie Callender's*), 7.5 oz. 300
parmigiana (*Marie Callender's* Multi-Serve), 8 oz. 320

Rockfish, meat only, baked, broiled, or microwaved, 4 oz. 137

Roe (see also "Caviar"):
raw, 1 tbsp. 22
baked, broiled, or microwaved, 4 oz. 231

Roll (see also "Biscuit"), 1 roll, except as noted:
brown and serve (*Pepperidge Farm* Hearth), 3 rolls 150
brown and serve, club (*Pepperidge Farm*) 120
brown and serve, French (*Pepperidge Farm* 3) 240
crescent, butter (*Pepperidge Farm* Heat & Serve) 110
dinner (*Pepperidge Farm* Country Style), 3 rolls 150
dinner, all varieties (*Awrey's*), 2 rolls, 1.6 oz. 110
dinner, finger or parke house (*Pepperidge Farm*), 3 rolls 150
dinner, potato (*Pepperidge Farm* Deli Classic) 80
French (*Pepperidge Farm*) 100
French, 7 grain (*Pepperidge Farm* 9) 80
French, sourdough (*Pepperidge Farm*) 100
golden twist (*Pepperidge Farm* Heat & Serve) 110
hamburger (*Pepperidge Farm*) 130

Roll ***(cont.)***
hoagie (*Awrey's*) 230
hoagie, all varieties (*Pepperidge Farm/Pepperidge Farm* Deli Classic) 200
hot dog, Dijon or plain (*Pepperidge Farm*) 140
kaiser or onion (*Arnold August Bros.*) 160
party (*Pepperidge Farm* 20), 5 rolls 170
sandwich (*Pepperidge Farm* Hearty) 230
sandwich, multigrain or onion (*Pepperidge Farm*) 150
sandwich, potato (*Pepperidge Farm*) 160
sandwich, sesame seed (*Pepperidge Farm*) 140
sandwich, sourdough (*Pepperidge Farm*) 170
Roll, frozen or refrigerated:
(*Rich's* Homestyle), 2 rolls 150
butterflake (*Pillsbury*), 1 roll 130
crescent (*Pillsbury*), 2 rolls 200
crescent, cheese (*Pillsbury*), 2 rolls 210
garlic and cheese (*Pepperidge Farm*), 1 roll 130
Roll, mix, hot:
(*Dromedary*), 1/16 pkg. 100
(*Pillsbury*), 1/15 pkg.* 130
Roll, sweet (see also "Bun, honey" and "Danish"), 1 piece:
cinnamon (*Hostess*) 220
pecan (*Little Debbie Pecan Spinwheels*) 220
Roll, sweet, frozen or refrigerated, 1 piece:
apple cinnamon or cinnamon raisin, with icing (*Pillsbury*) 140
caramel or iced orange (*Pillsbury*) 170
cinnamon (*Pepperidge Farm*) 250
cinnamon, with icing (*Pillsbury*) 140
Roman beans, canned (*Goya*), 1/2 cup 90
Rotini dishes, mix, dry:
mushroom sauce (*Knorr*), 2/3 cup 250
primavera (*Lipton* Pasta & Sauce), 1/2 pkg. 240
Roughy, orange, meat only, baked, broiled, or microwaved, 4 oz. 101
Roy Rogers, 1 serving:
breakfast dishes:
bagel, plain or cinnamon raisin 300

Big Country Breakfast Platter, with bacon 740
Big Country Breakfast Platter, with ham 710
Big Country Breakfast Platter, with sausage 920
biscuit, plain 390
biscuit, *Cinnamon 'N' Raisin* 370
biscuit, bacon 420
biscuit, bacon and egg 470
biscuit, ham and cheese 450
biscuit, ham and egg 460
biscuit, ham, egg, and cheese 500
biscuit, sausage 510
biscuit, sausage and egg 560
sourdough, ham, egg, and cheese 480
hash rounds 230
pancakes, plain, 3 pieces 280
pancakes, 3 pieces, with 2 strips bacon 350
pancakes, 3 pieces, with 1 sausage 430

sandwiches:
bacon cheeseburger 490
bacon cheeseburger, sourdough 730
cheeseburger 300
cheeseburger, ¼ lb. 470
chicken, grilled 340
chicken, grilled, sourdough 500
chicken fillet 500
Fisherman's Fillet 490
hamburger 260
hamburger, ¼ lb. 430
roast beef 260

chicken, fried:
breast 370
leg 170
thigh 330
wing 200

¼ Roy's Roaster:
dark meat 490
dark or white meat, skin off 190
white meat 500

chicken nuggets, 6 pieces 290

Roy Rogers (cont.)
chicken nuggets, 9 pieces 460
salads:
chicken, grilled 120
garden 190
side salad 140
potatoes:
baked 130
baked, with margarine 240
baked, with margarine and sour cream 300
fries, regular 350
fries, large 430
mashed, 5 oz. 92
gravy for mashed 20
sides:
baked beans, 5 oz. 160
coleslaw, 5 oz. 295
corn bread 310
Rum runner mixer, frozen* (*Bacardi*), 8 fl. oz. 140
Rutabaga, fresh, boiled, drained, mashed, 1/2 cup 47
Rye flour (*Arrowhead Mills*), 1/4 cup 100
Rye-wheat flour (*Pillsbury* Bohemian Style), 1/4 cup 100

S

FOOD AND MEASURE	CALORIES
Sablefish, meat only:	
baked, broiled, or microwaved, 4 oz.	284
smoked, 4 oz.	291
Salad blend mix, fresh:	
Caesar (*Dole Salad-in-a-Minute*), 3.5 oz.	170
Oriental (*Dole Salad-in-a-Minute*), 3.5 oz.	110
spinach (*Dole Salad-in-a-Minute*), 3.5 oz.	180
Salad dressing, 2 tbsp.:	
all varieties (*Nasoya Vegi-Dressing*)	60
bacon and tomato (*Kraft*)	140
balsamic vinegar (*S&W* Vintage Lites)	35
berry vinaigrette, triple (*Knott's Berry Farm*)	40
blue cheese (*Kraft Roka*)	90
blue cheese (*Marie's* Salad Bar/Chunky Reduced Calorie)	100
blue cheese, chunky (*Marie's*)	180
blue cheese, chunky (*Wish-Bone*)	170
blue cheese, chunky (*Wish-Bone* Lite)	80
blue cheese, creamy (*Marie's* Low Fat)	30
blue cheese, vinaigrette (*Herb Magic*)	160
Caesar, creamy (*Seven Seas*)	140
Caesar, creamy, with cracked pepper (*Lawry's*)	130
Caesar, roasted garlic (*Knott's Berry Farm*)	140
Caesar, with olive oil (*Wish-Bone*)	100
Caesar, with olive oil (*Wish-Bone* Lite)	60
Caesar, ranch (*Kraft*)	140
chicken salad, Oriental (*Knotts Berry Farm*)	130
citrus vinaigrette (*Knott's Berry Farm* California)	40
coleslaw (*Marie's*)	150
cucumber, creamy (*Herb Magic*)	15
Dijon vinaigrette (*Wish-Bone* Classic Lite)	60
French (*Kraft Catalina/Catalina* Honey)	140
French (*Nalley*)	110
French (*Wish-Bone*)	120

Salad dressing *(cont.)*
French, sweet 'n spicy (*Wish-Bone*) 130
French, tangy (*Marie's*) 130
French, true vinaigrette (*Herb Magic*) 170
fruit salad (*Knott's Berry Farm*) 70
fruit vinaigrette, Island (*Knott's Berry Farm*) 45
garden, zesty (*Kraft Salsa*) 70
garlic, roasted, creamy (*Wish-Bone*) 140
garlic, roasted, creamy (*Wish-Bone* Fat Free) 40
green goddess (*Seven Seas*) 120
herb vinaigrette, zesty (*Marie's* Fat Free) 30
herbs and spices (*Seven Seas*) 120
honey Dijon (*Wish-Bone*) 130
honey mustard (*Knott's Berry Farm*) 130
honey mustard (*Marie's*) 160
honey mustard (*Nally*) 130
Italian (*Herb Magic*) 10
Italian (*Kraft* Presto) 140
Italian (*Ott's* Zesty) 90
Italian (*Wish-Bone* Classic House) 140
Italian (*Wish-Bone/Wish-Bone Robusto*) 100
Italian, cheese, two (*Seven Seas*) 70
Italian, creamy (*Kraft*) 110
Italian, creamy (*Wish-Bone*) 100
Italian, creamy (*Wish-Bone* Lite) 60
Italian, garlic, creamy (*Marie's*) 180
Italian, garlic, creamy (*Marie's* Reduced Calorie) 90
Italian, herb, creamy (*Marie's* Low Fat) 30
Italian, olive oil (*Wish-Bone* Classic) 70
mango–key lime or Oriental rice wine vinegar (*S&W*
    Vintage Lites) 30
mayonnaise type, see "Mayonnaise"
(*Ott's* Famous Original) 80
Parmesan, creamy (*Marie's* Low Fat) 35
peppercorn, ground (*Knott's Berry Farm*) 160
poppyseed (*Herb Magic*) 170
poppyseed (*Knott's Berry Farm*) 120
poppyseed (*Marie's*) 150
potato salad (*Best Foods/Hellmann's One Step*) 160

potato salad (*Best Foods/Hellmann's One Step* 1/3 Less Fat) 110
ranch (*Herb Magic*) 15
ranch (*Marie's* Salad Bar Reduced Calorie) 90
ranch (*Ott's* Buttermilk) 140
ranch (*Wish-Bone*) 160
ranch, buttermilk or Parmesan (*Marie's*) 180
ranch, creamy (*Marie's* Reduced Calorie) 100
ranch, zesty (*Marie's* Low Fat) 30
raspberry blush vinegar (*S&W* Vintage Lites) 40
raspberry vinaigrette (*Knott's Berry Farm* Low Fat) 50
raspberry vinaigrette, zesty (*Marie's* Fat Free) 35
red or white wine vinegar, with herbs (*S&W* Vintage Lites) 40
red wine vinegar and oil (*Seven Seas*) 110
red or white wine vinaigrette, zesty (*Marie's* Fat Free) . . . 40
Russian (*Kraft*) 130
Russian (*Wish-Bone*) 110
Santa Fe or Sierra (*Wish-Bone*) 150
sour cream and dill (*Marie's*) 190
sweet and sour (*Herb Magic*) 35
sweet and sour (*Old Dutch*) 50
Thousand Island (*Marie's*) 240
Thousand Island (*Marie's* Salad Bar) 170
Thousand Island (*Wish-Bone*) 130
Thousand Island, with bacon (*Kraft*) 120
tomato, sun-dried, vinaigrette (*Knotts Berry Farm*) 100
tuna salad (*Best Foods/Hellmann's One Step*) 140

Salad dressing mix, 2 tbsp.*:
Caesar or honey mustard (*Good Seasons*) 150
cheese garlic, garlic and herbs, or Mexican spice (*Good Seasons*) 140
Italian, regular or zesty (*Good Seasons*) 140
Oriental sesame or mild Italian (*Good Seasons*) 150
ranch or farm-style buttermilk (*Good Seasons*) 120

Salad toppers, all varieties (*Pepperidge Farm*), 1 tbsp. . . . 35

Salami:
beef (*Hebrew National*), 2 oz. 170
beef (*Hebrew National* Lean), 2 oz. 90

Salami ***(cont.)***

beef (*Oscar Mayer* Machiach), 2 slices, 1.6 oz. 120
cooked (*Boar's Head*), 2 oz. 130
cotto (*Oscar Mayer*), 2 slices, 1.6 oz. 110
cotto, beef (*Oscar Mayer*), 2 slices, 1.6 oz. 90
dry or hard (*Boar's Head*), 1 oz. 110
dry or hard (*Hormel Homeland/Sandwich Maker*), 1 oz. 110
Genoa (*Boar's Head*), 2 oz. 180
Genoa (*Di Lusso/San Remo Brand*), 1 oz. 120
Genoa (*Hormel Pillow Pack/Sandwich Maker*), 1 oz. . . . 120

Salmon, fresh, meat only, 4 oz.:

Atlantic, farmed, baked, broiled, or microwaved 234
Atlantic, wild, baked, broiled, or microwaved 206
Chinook, baked, broiled, or microwaved 262
chum, baked, broiled, or microwaved 175
coho, farmed, baked, broiled, or microwaved 202
coho, wild, baked, broiled, or microwaved 158
coho, wild, boiled, poached, or steamed 209
pink, baked, broiled, or microwaved 169
sockeye, baked, broiled, or microwaved 245

Salmon, canned:

chum or coho (*Peter Pan*), 1/4 cup 90
king (*Peter Pan*), 1/4 cup 140
Norwegian fillet (*Abelvaer*), 3 oz. 170
pink, skinless fillet (*Chicken of the Sea*), 2 oz. 60
pink, skinless fillet (*Peter Pan*), 1/4 cup 90
red (*Peter Pan*), 1/4 cup 110
red, blueback (*Rubinstein's*), 1/4 cup 110
red, sockeye (*S&W*), 1/4 cup 110

Salmon, frozen, 4 oz.:

chum, fillet or steak (*Peter Pan*) 130
coho, fillet (*Peter Pan*) 160

Salmon, refrigerated, Alaska, boneless and skinless:

burger (*Salmon Chef*), 3-oz. burger 80
cuts (*Salmon Chef*), 5-oz. piece 110
cuts, in dill sorrel chive marinade (*Salmon Chef*),
5-oz. piece 140
kabob (*Salmon Chef*), 3.3-oz. kabob 100

kabob, teriyaki sesame marinade (*Salmon Chef*), 3.3-oz. kabob 110
loin (*Salmon Chef*), 2 pieces, 4 oz. 110
loin, in chili cilantro marinade (*Salmon Chef*), 2 pieces, 4 oz. 130
tenderloin (*Salmon Chef*), 6-oz. piece 110
tenderloin, sweet pepper–sage marinade (*Salmon Chef*), 6-oz. piece 160

Salmon, smoked:
Chinook, regular or lox, 4 oz. 133
lox or Nova (*Vita*), 2 oz. 50

Salmon, smoked, spread (*Vita*), ¼ cup, 2 oz. 180

Salsa (see also "Picante sauce"), 2 tbsp., except as noted:
(*Kaukauna* Extra Chunky) 14
(*La Victoria* Victoria) 5
(*Marie's* Tomato) 10
(*Pace* Thick & Chunky) 10
all varieties (*Hunt's* Alfresco Homestyle) 10
all varieties (*Hunt's* Homestyle) 30
all varieties (*La Victoria* Jalapeña/Ranchera/Suprema/ Thick N Chunky) 10
all varieties (*Rosarita*) 10
all varieties (*S&W* Ready-Cut), ¼ cup 20
all varieties (*Tostitos*) 15
garlic, roasted (*Marie's*) .10
green chili (*La Victoria*) .10
hot (*Guiltless Gourmet*) 10
hot or mild (*Sun-Vista*) 5
hot or mild (*Heluva* Good Thick & Chunky) 10
picante (*Old Dutch*) 10

Salsa seasoning (*Lawry's*), ½ tsp. 5

Salsify, boiled, drained, sliced, ½ cup 46

Sandwich dressing (*Vlasic Sandwich Zesters*), 2 tbsp.:
bell pepper salsa, garden onion, or jalapeño salsa 15
Italian tomato or mushroom and onion 10

Sandwich sauce, ¼ cup:
(*Hunt's Manwich* Original) 30
(*Hunt's Manwich* Thick & Chunky) 45

Sandwich sauce *(cont.)*
barbecue or bold (*Hunt's Manwich/Hunt's Manwich* Bold) . 60
Mexican (*Hunt's Manwich*) 25
Sloppy Joe (*Del Monte* Original) 50
Sloppy Joe, hickory flavor (*Del Monte*) 60
Sandwich sauce seasoning mix, Sloppy Joe (*Lawry's*), 1 tsp. 15
Sandwich spread (see also "Sandwich sauce" and specific listings):
meat (*Oscar Mayer* Sandwich Spread), 2 oz. 130
relish (*Blue Plate*), 1 tbsp. 75
relish (*Hellmann's*), 1 tbsp. 50
Sangria juice (*After the Fall* Sangria de la Noche), 8 fl. oz. 125
Sapodilla, 1 medium, 3″ × 2½″ 140
Sapote, 1 medium, 11.2 oz. 301
Sardine, fresh, see "Herring"
Sardine, canned:
Atlantic, in oil, drained, 2 medium, 3″ long 50
in lemon or spiced (*Goya*), ¼ cup 120
in olive oil, drained, Norway brisling (*S&W*), 3¾-oz. can 160
in olive oil, drained, skinless, boneless (*S&W*), 3¾-oz. can 100
in olive oil or tomato sauce (*Goya*), ¼ cup 130
in soy oil, drained, skinless, boneless (*King Oscar*), 1.9 oz., 3 pieces 120
in tomato sauce (*Del Monte*), 2 oz., ½ fish with sauce . . . 80
Sauerkraut:
(*S&W*), 2 tbsp. 5
(*Stokely*), ½ cup 25
Bavarian style (*Stokely*), ½ cup 35
sweet and sour (*Stokely*), ½ cup 80
Sauerkraut juice (*S&W*), 10-oz. can 35
Sausage (see also "Chicken sausage" and "Turkey sausage"), cooked:
(*Hormel Special Recipe*), 1-oz. link 111
(*Hormel Special Recipe*), 1.5-oz. patty 178
beef, smoked (*Oscar Mayer* Smokies), 1.5-oz. link 120
brown and serve (*Little Sizzlers*), 3 links 230

brown and serve (*Little Sizzlers*), 2 patties 190
dinner, Italian or sandwich (*Jones Dairy Farm*), 1 link or patty 140
pickled, smoked or hot (*Hormel*), 6 links, 2 oz. 140
pork (*Oscar Mayer*), 2 links 170
pork, hot and spicy or regular (*Little Sizzlers*), 3 links . . 180
pork, all flavors (*Jones Dairy Farm* Golden Brown), 2 links 190
pork, light (*Jones Dairy Farm* Golden Brown Lite), 2 links 110
pork patty (*Jones Dairy Farm* All Natural), 1 patty 130
pork patty (*Little Sizzlers*), 2 patties 210
pork roll, regular or hot (*Jones Dairy Farm* All Natural), 2 oz. 230
smoked (*Boar's Head*), 4.5 oz. 400
smoked (*John Morrell* Bun Size), 3-oz. link 270
smoked (*Oscar Mayer* Little Smokies), 6 links, 2 oz. . . . 170
smoked, cheese or regular (*Oscar Mayer* Smokie Links), 1.5-oz. link 130
smoked, hot (*Boar's Head*), 3.2 oz. 280
Sausage biscuit, frozen:
(*Hormel Quick Meal*), 1 piece 350
(*Weight Watchers*), 3 oz. 230
with cheese (*Hormel Quick Meal*), 1 piece 410
with egg (*Hormel Quick Meal*), 1 piece 390
with egg, cheese (*Swanson Great Starts*), 1 pkg. 490
Sausage gravy mix (*Durkee/French's*), ¼ cup* 35
Sausage hash, canned (*Mary Kitchen*), 1 cup 410
Sausage stick, 1 piece, except as noted:
(*Tombstone* Beef/Snappy Sticks) 110
beef (*Boar's Head*), .6 oz. 100
beef or summer sausage (*Old Dutch*), 1 oz. 110
beef (*Rustlers Roundup* Jerky) 30
beef (*Tombstone* Jerky) 35
hot (*Rustlers Roundup* Flamin') 40
smoked (*Rustlers Roundup* Steak Stick) 60
smoked, mild or spicy (*Slim Jim*), 1.4-oz. box 210
spicy (*Rustlers Roundup*) 50
Scallop, meat only, raw, 4 oz. 100

"Scallop" vegetarian, canned (*Loma Linda Tender Bits*), 6 pieces 110
Scallop entree, fried, frozen (*Mrs. Paul's*), 12 pieces . . . 200
Scallop squash:
boiled, drained, sliced, 1/2 cup 14
boiled, drained, mashed, 1/2 cup 19
Scrapple (*Jones Dairy Farm*), 2 oz. 120
Scrod, fresh, see "Cod" (Atlantic)
Scup, meat only, baked, broiled, or microwaved, 4 oz. . . 153
Sea bass, meat only, baked, broiled, or microwaved, 4 oz. 141
Sea trout, meat only, baked, broiled, or microwaved, 4 oz. 151
Seafood sauce (see also specific listings):
(*Bookbinder's*), 1/4 cup 70
(*Crosse & Blackwell*), 1/4 cup 110
(*Heinz*), 1/4 cup 60
(*Heluva* Good), 1/4 cup 40
(*Maull's*), 2 tbsp. 45
(*Sauceworks*), 1/4 cup 60
(*S&W*), 1 tsp. 20
Seasoning and coating mix (see also specific listings):
country mild (*Shake 'n Bake*), 1/8 pkt. 35
glaze, tangy honey or honey mustard (*Shake 'n Bake*), 1/8 pkt. 45
Italian herb (*Shake 'n Bake*), 1/8 pkt. 40
Seaweed:
agar, flakes or bar (*Eden*), 1 tbsp. 10
arame or hiziki (*Eden*), 1/2 cup 30
kombu (*Eden*), 1/2 of 7" piece 10
nori (*Eden*), 1 sheet 10
spirulina, dried, 1 oz. 82
wakame (*Eden/Eden* Flakes), 1/2 cup 25
Semolina flour, mix (*Arrowhead Mills*), 1/2 cup 240
Sesame butter (see also "Sesame paste") (*Roaster Fresh*), 1 oz. 168
Sesame paste (see also "Tahini"), from whole seeds, 1 tbsp. 95

Sesame seeds:
whole, brown (*Arrowhead Mills*), 1/4 cup 200
kernels, decorticated (*Arrowhead Mills*), 1/4 cup 210
kernels, toasted, 1 oz. 161
Shad, American, meat only, baked, broiled, or
microwaved, 4 oz. 286
Shallot:
fresh or stored, chopped, 1 tbsp. 7
freeze-dried, 1 tbsp. 3
Shark, meat only, raw, 4 oz. 148
Shellie beans, canned (*Stokely*), 1/2 cup 45
Shells, pasta, stuffed, entree, frozen:
(*Celentano*), 10 oz. 400
(*Celentano* Great Choice), 10 oz. 250
broccoli (*Celentano* Great Choice), 10 oz. 190
Florentine (*Celentano*), 10 oz. 240
Sherbet (see also "Ice" and "Sorbet"):
orange (*Carnation* Cup), 3 fl. oz. 90
orange, Swiss (*Edy's*), 1/2 cup 150
pink lemonade, tangerine, or tropical (*Edy's*), 1/2 cup . . . 130
strawberry kiwi (*Edy's*), 1/2 cup 120
Shortening, vegetable, regular or butter flavor (*Crisco*),
1 tbsp. 110
Shrimp, meat only:
boiled or steamed, 4 oz. 112
boiled or steamed, 4 large 22
Shrimp, canned, deveined, small or medium (*S&W*),
1/4 cup 45
"Shrimp," imitation, frozen, jumbo (*Captain Jac Shrimp
Tasties*), 3 pieces, 3 oz. 80
Shrimp cocktail (*Vita*), 4-oz. jar 110
Shrimp entree, canned, chow mein (*La Choy* Bi-Pack),
1 cup 55
Shrimp entree, frozen:
batter, beer (*Gorton's*), 6 pieces 250
breaded (*Gorton's* Original), 6 pieces 230
breaded (*Mrs. Paul's* Special Recipe), 1 pkg. 350
breaded, with angel-hair pasta (*Marie Callender's*), 1 cup 300
breaded, butterfly (*Van de Kamp's*), 7 shrimp 280

Shrimp entree, frozen *(cont.)*
breaded, scampi (*Gorton's*), 6 pieces 250
breaded, whole (*Van de Kamp's*), 4 oz., 7 shrimp 240
marinara (*Healthy Choice*), 10.5 oz. 220
marinara (*Smart Ones*), 9 oz. 200
popcorn, breaded (*Gorton's*), 1 cup, 3.2 oz. 260
popcorn, breaded (*Van de Kamp's*), 4 oz., 20 pieces . . . 270
popcorn, breaded, garlic and herb (*Gorton's*), 1¼ cups, 3.5 oz. 270
and vegetables (*Healthy Choice*), 12.5 oz. 270
Shrimp entree mix, Creole (*Luzianne*), ⅕ pkg. 150
Shrimp sauce (*Crosse & Blackwell*), ¼ cup 110
Sloppy Joe entree, frozen (*Swanson Fun Feast*), 1 pkg. 290
Sloppy Joe sauce, see "Sandwich sauce"
Smelt, rainbow, meat only, baked, broiled, or microwaved, 4 oz. 141
Snack chips and crisps (see also specific listings):
apple cinnamon or raspberry (*Crunchwells Crumpet Chips*), 1 oz. 110
cheddar (*Old Dutch Multicrisps*), 1 oz. 130
mixed (*Terra* Chips), 1 oz. 140
onion (*Funyons*), 1 oz. 140
onion, French (*Old Dutch Multicrisps*), 1 oz. 128
Parmesan garlic or barbecue (*Crunchwells Crumpet Chips*), 1 oz. 100
Snack mix, ½ cup, except as noted:
(*Cheez-It*) 140
(*Old Dutch* Party Mix), ⅔ cup, 1.1 oz. 150
(*Pepperidge Farm* Lightly Seasoned/Goldfish) 170
cheddar, zesty (*Pepperidge Farm* Goldfish) 180
honey mustard and onion or extra nutty (*Pepperidge Farm*) 180
Snapper, meat only, baked, broiled, or microwaved, 4 oz. 145
Snow pea, see "Peas, edible-podded"
Snow pea sprouts (*Jonathan's*), 1 cup, 3.5 oz. 40
Soft drinks, carbonated:
all varieties (*R.W. Knudsen Fruit TeaZer*/Spritzer), 12 fl. oz. 110

all varieties (*Santa Cruz* Sparkling), 12 fl. oz. 150
almond, amaretto (*After the Fall*), 12 fl. oz. 150
apple, spiced (*Natural Brew*), 12 fl. oz. 170
berry (*After the Fall* Berrymeister), 12 fl. oz. 160
birch beer (*Canada Dry*), 8 fl. oz. 110
cafe mocha (*Natural Brew*), 12 fl. oz. 150
(*Canada Dry* Cactus Cooler/*Hi-Spot*), 8 fl. oz. 110
cherry (*Sundrop*), 12 fl. oz. 180
cherry, amaretto (*Natural Brew*), 12 fl. oz. 160
cherry, black (*Shasta*), 12 fl. oz. 170
cherry, French (*Snapple*), 8 fl. oz. 120
cherry, wild (*Canada Dry*), 8 fl. oz. 110
cherry-lime (*Spree*), 12 fl. oz. 170
cherry–lime rickey (*Snapple*), 8 fl. oz. 110
citrus (*Canada Dry* Half & Half), 8 fl. oz. 110
club soda or seltzer (*Canada Dry/Schweppes*), 12 fl. oz. . . .0
cola (*Coca-Cola* Classic), 8 fl. oz. 100
cola (*Pepsi/Crystal Pepsi*), 12 fl. oz. 150
cola (*Shasta*), 12 fl. oz. 170
cola, cherry (*Shasta*), 12 fl. oz. 160
cola, cherry, wild (*Pepsi*), 12 fl. oz. 160
cola, ginseng (*Natural Brew*), 12 fl. oz. 170
collins mixer (*Canada Dry/Schweppes*), 8 fl. oz. 100
cranberry (*Shasta*), 12 fl. oz. 180
cream (*A&W*), 8 fl. oz. 110
cream (*Hires*), 12 fl. oz. 180
cream (*Shasta*), 12 fl. oz. 190
cream, vanilla (*Canada Dry*), 8 fl. oz. 120
cream, vanilla (*Natural Brew*), 12 fl. oz. 170
cream, vanilla (*Snapple*), 8 fl. oz. 130
(*Doc Shasta*), 12 fl. oz. 160
(*Dr Pepper*), 12 fl. oz. 160
fruit punch (*Shasta*), 12 fl. oz. 200
ginger ale (*Canada Dry/Schweppes*), 8 fl. oz. 90
ginger ale (*Canada Dry* Golden), 8 fl. oz. 100
ginger ale (*Natural Brew* Outrageous), 12 fl. oz. 170
ginger ale (*Shasta*), 12 fl. oz. 130
ginger ale, cranberry or lemon (*Canada Dry*), 8 fl. oz. . . .90
ginger ale, grape or raspberry (*Schweppes*), 8 fl. oz. . . . 100

Soft drinks *(cont.)*

ginger beer (*Schweppes*), 8 fl. oz. 100
grape (*Canada Dry* Concord), 8 fl. oz. 120
grape (*Schweppes*), 8 fl. oz. 130
grape (*Shasta*), 12 fl. oz. 190
grapefruit (*Schweppes*), 8 fl. oz. 110
grapefruit (*Shasta* Ruby Red), 12 fl. oz. 190
grapefruit (*Wink*), 8 fl. oz. 130
kiwi-strawberry (*Shasta*), 12 fl. oz. 170
kiwi-strawberry (*Snapple*), 8 fl. oz. 130
kiwi-strawberry or peach vanilla (*After the Fall*), 12 fl. oz. 170
lemon, bitter or sour (*Schweppes*), 8 fl. oz. 110
lemon-lime (*Schweppes*), 8 fl. oz. 100
lemon-lime (*Spree*), 12 fl. oz. 170
lime (*After the Fall* Caribbean), 12 fl. oz. 170
lime (*Canada Dry* Island), 8 fl. oz. 140
lime-lemon (*Shasta Twist*), 12 fl. oz. 150
mango or mandarin pineapple (*After the Fall* Hawaiian),
12 fl. oz. 180
(*Mountain Dew*), 12 fl. oz. 170
orange (*Crush*), 12 fl. oz. 200
orange (*Orangina*), 10 fl. oz. 120
orange (*Shasta*), 12 fl. oz. 200
passion fruit (*Snapple*), 8 fl. oz. 120
peach (*Shasta*), 12 fl. oz. 170
peach (*Snapple* Melba), 8 fl. oz. 120
pineapple (*Shasta*), 12 fl. oz. 200
pineapple-orange (*Shasta*), 12 fl. oz. 180
raspberry (*Snapple* Royal), 8 fl. oz. 120
raspberry creme (*Shasta*), 12 fl. oz. 170
raspberry or vanilla bean (*After the Fall*), 12 fl. oz. 170
red (*Shasta*), 12 fl. oz. 170
root beer (*Hires*), 12 fl. oz. 180
root beer (*Mug*), 12 fl. oz. 160
root beer (*Shasta*), 12 fl. oz. 170
root beer (*Snapple* Tru), 8 fl. oz. 110
(*7Up/7Up* Cherry), 12 fl. oz. 160
sour mixer (*Canada Dry*), 8 fl. oz. 90
strawberry (*Shasta*), 12 fl. oz. 190

strawberry-peach (*Shasta*), 12 fl. oz. 170
(*Sundrop*), 12 fl. oz. 200
tonic (*Schweppes*), 8 fl. oz. 90
Sole, fresh, see "Flatfish"
Sole, frozen (*Van de Kamp's* Natural), 4 oz. 110
Sole entree, frozen, breaded (*Mrs. Paul's*Premium),
1 fillet 250
Sopressata (*Boar's Head Cinghiale* Mini), 1 oz. 100
Sorbet (see also "Ice" and "Sherbet"), ½ cup:
(*Ben & Jerry's Doonesbury*) 130
chocolate, lemon, or orange peach mango (*Tofutti*) 90
coffee, raspberry, or strawberry (*Tofutti*) 80
and cream, orange (*Häagen-Dazs*) 200
and cream, raspberry (*Häagen-Dazs*) 190
mocha or piña colada (*Ben & Jerry's*) 140
pink lemonade or purple passion (*Ben & Jerry's*) 120
strawberry kiwi (*Ben & Jerry's*) 100
Soup, canned, ready-to-serve, 1 cup, except as noted:
bean (*Grandma Brown's*) 190
bean, salsa (*Campbell's* Home Cookin') 160
bean with bacon and ham (*Campbell's* Microwave),
1 container 180
bean and ham (*Campbell's* Chunky) 190
bean and ham (*Campbell's* Home Cookin') 180
bean and ham (*Healthy Choice*) 185
beans and rice Creole (*Campbell's* Chunky) 210
beef, chunky (*Campbell's* Microwave), 1 container 210
beef, pasta (*Campbell's* Chunky) 150
beef, potato (*Healthy Choice*) 120
beef, vegetable, country (*Campbell's* Chunky) 160
beef broth (*Swanson*) 20
beef Stroganoff (*Campbell's* Chunky), 10¾-oz. can 310
borscht (*Gold's*) 70
broccoli cheese (*Campbell's* Chunky) 200
chicken (*Campbell's* Chunky Old Fashioned) 130
chicken, cream of (*Campbell's* Home Cookin') 210
chicken, hearty (*Healthy Choice*) 130
chicken broth (*Campbell's Healthy Request*) 20
chicken broth (*Swanson*) 30

Soup, canned, ready-to-serve *(cont.)*
chicken corn chowder (*Campbell's Healthy Request*) . . . 140
chicken mushroom chowder (*Campbell's* Chunky) 210
chicken noodle (*Campbell's* Chunky Classic) 130
chicken noodle (*Campbell's* Home Cookin') 100
chicken noodle (*Campbell's* Microwave), 1 container 90
chicken noodle (*Healthy Choice* Old Fashioned) 140
chicken noodle, chunky (*Campbell's* Microwave),
1 container 160
chicken noodle, creamy (*Campbell's* Chunky) 210
chicken noodle, hearty (*Campbell's Healthy Request*) . . . 160
chicken noodle, with mushroom (*Campbell's* Chunky) . . 120
chicken pasta (*Healthy Choice*) 120
chicken rice (*Campbell's* Chunky) 140
chicken rice (*Campbell's* Home Cookin') 110
chicken rice (*Campbell's* Microwave), 1 container 120
chicken rice (*Campbell's Healthy Request*) 100
chicken with rice (*Healthy Choice*) 110
chicken vegetable (*Campbell's* Chunky) 90
chicken vegetable (*Campbell's* Home Cookin') 130
chicken vegetable, hearty (*Campbell's Healthy Request*) 120
chicken vegetable, nuggets (*Campbell's* Chunky) 150
chili beef, with beans (*Campbell's* Chunky) 230
chili beef, with beans (*Campbell's* Microwave),
1 container 180
chili beef, with beans (*Healthy Choice*) 165
clam chowder, Manhattan (*Campbell's* Chunky) 130
clam chowder, New England (*Campbell's* Chunky) 240
clam chowder, New England (*Campbell's Healthy Request*) 120
clam chowder, New England (*Campbell's* Home Cookin') 210
clam chowder, New England (*Campbell's* Microwave),
1 container 200
clam chowder, New England (*Healthy Choice*) 125
clam chowder, New England, chunky (*Campbell's* Microwave), 1 container 290
corn chowder (*Campbell's* Chunky) 250
corn chowder, chicken (*Healthy Choice*) 175
egg flower or hot and sour (*Rice Road*) 90

lentil (*Healthy Choice*) 145
lentil, hearty (*Campbell's* Home Cookin') 130
minestrone (*Campbell's* Chunky) 140
minestrone (*Healthy Choice*) 110
minestrone, hearty (*Campbell's Healthy Request*) 120
minestrone, Tuscany (*Campbell's* Home Cookin') 160
mushroom, cream of (*Campbell's* Home Cookin') 170
mushroom, cream of (*Healthy Choice*) 75
mushroom and rice (*Campbell's* Home Cookin') 80
Oriental broth (*Swanson*) 15
pasta, Chinese (*Rice Road*) 70
pea, split (*Campbell's* Low Sodium), 10¾-oz. can 240
pea, split (*Grandma Brown's*) 210
pea, split, with ham (*Campbell's* Chunky) 190
pea, split, with ham (*Campbell's* Home Cookin'/*Healthy Request*) 170
pea, split, with ham (*Healthy Choice*) 155
penne, zesty (*Campbell's Healthy Request*) 90
pepper steak (*Campbell's* Chunky) 140
sirloin burger, chunky (*Campbell's* Microwave), 1 container 210
sirloin burger, with vegetable (*Campbell's* Chunky) 190
steak and potato (*Campbell's* Chunky) 160
tomato, garden (*Campbell's* Home Cookin'), 10¾-oz. can 150
tomato, garden (*Healthy Choice*) 105
tomato, vegetable (*Campbell's Healthy Request*) 120
turkey with wild rice (*Healthy Choice*) 100
turkey with wild rice, vegetable (*Campbell's Healthy Request*) 120
vegetable, regular or hearty, with pasta (*Campbell's* Chunky) 130
vegetable (*Campbell's* Microwave), 1 container 100
vegetable (*Campbell's Healthy Request*) 120
vegetable, country (*Campbell's* Home Cookin') 110
vegetable, country (*Healthy Choice*) 105
vegetable, garden (*Healthy Choice*) 130
vegetable, harborside (*Campbell's* Home Cookin') 80
vegetable, hearty (*Campbell's Healthy Request*) 100
vegetable, Italian (*Campbell's* Home Cookin') 100

Soup, canned, ready-to-serve *(cont.)*
vegetable, Mediterranean (*Campbell's* Chunky) 140
vegetable, Southwestern (*Campbell's* Home Cookin') . . . 130
vegetable, Southwestern (*Campbell's Healthy Request*) . . 140
vegetable beef (*Campbell's* Chunky) 150
vegetable beef (*Campbell's* Home Cookin') 120
vegetable beef (*Campbell's* Microwave), 1 container 90
vegetable beef (*Healthy Choice*) 130
vegetable beef, hearty (*Campbell's Healthy Request*) . . . 140
vegetable broth (*Swanson*) 20
Soup, canned, condensed, undiluted, ½ cup:
asparagus, cream of (*Campbell's*) 110
bean, with bacon (*Campbell's*) 180
bean, with bacon (*Campbell's Healthy Request*) 150
bean, black (*Campbell's*) 120
beef broth, double rich (*Campbell's*) 15
beef consommé (*Campbell's*) 25
beef noodle (*Campbell's*) 70
beef with vegetables, barley (*Campbell's*) 80
broccoli, cream of (*Campbell's Healthy Request*) 70
broccoli, potato or shrimp, cream of (*Campbell's*) 100
broccoli cheese (*Campbell's*) 110
celery, cream of (*Campbell's*) 110
celery, cream of (*Campbell's Healthy Request*) 70
cheese, cheddar (*Campbell's*) 130
cheese, nacho (*Campbell's*) 140
chicken, alphabet, with vegetables (*Campbell's*) 80
chicken, broth (*Campbell's*) 30
chicken, cream of (*Campbell's*) 130
chicken, cream of (*Campbell's Healthy Request*) 70
chicken, cream of, and broccoli (*Campbell's*) 120
chicken, cream of, and broccoli (*Campbell's Healthy Request*) 80
chicken, dumplings or noodle O's (*Campbell's*) 80
chicken, gumbo or noodle (*Campbell's*) 60
chicken, noodle (*Campbell's* Homestyle) 70
chicken, noodle (*Campbell's Healthy Request*) 70
chicken, noodle, creamy or creamy mushroom (*Campbell's*) 130

chicken, with rice, wild rice, or stars (*Campbell's*) 70
chicken, with rice (*Campbell's Healthy Request*) 60
chicken, won ton (*Campbell's*) 45
chicken vegetable (*Campbell's*) 80
chicken vegetable (*Campbell's Healthy Request*) 80
chicken vegetable, Southwestern (*Campbell's*) 110
chili beef, with beans (*Campbell's*) 170
clam chowder, Manhattan (*Campbell's*) 60
clam chowder, New England (*Campbell's*) 100
clam chowder, New England (*Doxsee*) 90
corn, golden (*Campbell's*) 120
minestrone (*Campbell's*) 100
minestrone or tomato (*Campbell's Healthy Request*) 90
mushroom, beefy (*Campbell's*) 70
mushroom, cream of (*Campbell's*) 110
mushroom, cream of (*Campbell's Healthy Request/*
Reduced Fat) 70
mushroom, golden (*Campbell's*) 80
noodle, curly, chicken broth (*Campbell's*) 80
noodle, double, chicken broth (*Campbell's*) 100
noodle and ground beef or pepperpot (*Campbell's*) 100
onion, creamy, or cream of Mexican pepper (*Campbell's*) 110
onion, French, with beef stock (*Campbell's*) 70
oyster stew (*Campbell's*) 90
pea, green, or split pea with ham and bacon
(*Campbell's*) 180
Scotch broth (*Campbell's*) 80
tomato, regular or Italian with basil and oregano
(*Campbell's*) 100
tomato, cream of (*Campbell's* Homestyle) 110
tomato bisque (*Campbell's*) 130
tomato fiesta (*Campbell's*) 70
tomato rice (*Campbell's* Old Fashioned) 120
turkey noodle, turkey vegetable, or vegetable
(*Campbell's*) 80
vegetable (*Campbell's* Homestyle/Old Fashioned) 70
vegetable, beef (*Campbell's/Campbell's Healthy Request*) . 80
vegetable, California style (*Campbell's*) 60
vegetable, hearty or regular (*Campbell's Healthy Request*) . 90

Soup, canned, condensed *(cont.)*
vegetable, hearty, with pasta (*Campbell's*) 90
vegetable, vegetarian (*Campbell's*) 70
Soup, canned, semi-condensed, undiluted, ⅔ cup:
bacon, lettuce, tomato, with chicken broth (*Pepperidge Farm*) 130
black bean with sherry (*Pepperidge Farm*) 120
broccoli, cream of (*Pepperidge Farm*) 90
chicken curry (*Pepperidge Farm*) 170
chicken with rice (*Pepperidge Farm*) 80
chicken with rice, with bacon and ham (*Campbell's*) . . . 150
clam chowder, Manhattan (*Pepperidge Farm*) 80
clam chowder, New England (*Pepperidge Farm*) 160
consommé Madrilene (*Pepperidge Farm*) 50
corn chowder (*Pepperidge Farm*) 140
crab (*Pepperidge Farm*) 80
gazpacho (*Pepperidge Farm*) 70
hunter's, with turkey and beef (*Pepperidge Farm*) 130
lobster bisque (*Pepperidge Farm*) 160
minestrone (*Pepperidge Farm*) 100
mushroom, shiitake (*Pepperidge Farm*) 80
onion, French (*Pepperidge Farm*) 50
oyster stew (*Pepperidge Farm*) 160
pea, green, with ham (*Pepperidge Farm*) 210
vichyssoise (*Pepperidge Farm*) 120
watercress (*Pepperidge Farm*) 80
Soup mix, dry:
barley vegetable, hearty (*Fantastic* Cup), 1.5 oz. 150
bean, black (*Bean Cuisine* Island), 1 serving 126
bean, black, hearty (*Fantastic Jumpin'* Cup), 2.2 oz. . . . 210
bean, black, Santa Fe (*Campbell's Soupsations*), 1 pkg. 250
bean, 5, hearty (*Fantastic* Cup), 2.3 oz. 230
bean, white (*Bean Cuisine* Provençal), 1 serving 103
bean and ham (*Hormel* Micro Cup), 1 pkg. 190
beef vegetable (*Hormel* Micro Cup), 7.5 oz. 90
broccoli-cheese, cheddar, creamy (*Fantastic* Cup), 1.5 oz. 130
broccoli-cheese, with ham (*Hormel* Micro Cup), 7.5 oz. 170
chicken (*Campbell's* Instant), 1 pkg. 130
chicken, noodle (*Campbell's* Soup/Recipe), 3 tbsp. 100

chicken, noodle or rice (*Hormel* Micro Cup), 7.5 oz. . . . 110
chicken, onion and rice (*Kettle Creations*), 1/4 pkg. 120
chicken, pasta and beans (*Kettle Creations*), 1/4 pkg. . . . 110
chili, hearty (*Fantastic Cha-Cha* Cup), 2.4 oz. 220
clam chowder, New England (*Hormel* Micro Cup), 7.5 oz. 130
corn chowder and potato, creamy (*Fantastic* Cup),
1.7 oz. 170
couscous with lentil, hearty (*Fantastic* Cup), 2.3 oz. 230
gumbo, New Orleans (*Campbell's Soupsations*), 1 pkg. . . 170
herb, golden, with lemon (*Lipton Recipe Secrets*),
2 tbsp. 35
herb, Italian, with tomato (*Lipton Recipe Secrets*),
2 tbsp. 40
herb with garlic, savory (*Lipton Recipe Secrets*), 1 tbsp. . 35
lentil, hearty (*Campbell's Soupsations*/Soup/Recipe),
1 pkg. 240
lentil, hearty (*Fantastic* Country Cup), 2.3 oz. 230
minestrone (*Kettle Creations*), 1/4 pkg. 110
minestrone, hearty (*Fantastic* Cup), 1.5 oz. 150
mushroom, beefy (*Lipton Recipe Secrets*), 2 tbsp. 35
mushroom, creamy (*Fantastic* Cup), 1.4 oz. 120
noodle, chicken free (*Fantastic* Cup), 1.5 oz. 140
noodle, extra (*Lipton Soup Secrets*), 3 tbsp. 90
noodle, all flavors (*Nissin Top Ramen*), 1.5 oz. 200
noodle, beef (*Campbell's* Instant), 1 pkg. 120
noodle, beef, crab, pork, or shrimp (*Nissin Cup Noodles*), 2.25 oz. 290
noodle, beef, onion (*Nissin Cup Noodles*), 2.25 oz. 280
noodle, chicken (*Lipton Soup Secrets*), 3 tbsp. 80
noodle, chicken, all flavors (*Nissin Cup Noodles*),
2.25 oz. 300
noodle, chicken, broth (*Campbell's* Instant), 1 pkg. 130
noodle, chicken, hearty (*Lipton Soup Secrets*), 1/4 cup . . . 80
noodle, lobster (*Nissin Cup Noodles*), 2.25 oz. 300
noodle, vegetable, curry (*Fantastic* Cup), 1.5 oz. 140
noodle, vegetable, egg, in broth (*Campbell's Soupsations*), 1 pkg. 150
noodle, vegetable, garden (*Nissin Cup Noodles*), 2.25 oz. 290
noodle, vegetable, hearty (*Campbell's* Instant), 1 pkg. . . 150

Soup mix *(cont.)*
noodle, vegetable, hearty (*Lipton Soup Secrets*), 3 tbsp. . 70
noodle, vegetable, miso (*Fantastic* Cup), 1.3 oz. 130
noodle, tomato (*Fantastic* Cup), 1.5 oz. 150
onion (*Campbell's* Soup/Recipe), 2 tbsp. 50
onion (*Lipton Recipe Secrets*), 1 tbsp. 20
onion, beefy (*Lipton Recipe Secrets*), 1 tbsp. 25
onion, golden (*Lipton Recipe Secrets*), 2 tbsp. 60
onion, mushroom (*Lipton Recipe Secrets*), 2 tbsp. 35
pasta, ruffle (*Lipton Soup Secrets*), 2 tbsp. 60
pasta and bean (*Kettle Creations*), 1/4 pkg. 130
pea, split, hearty (*Fantastic* Cup), 2 oz. 190
potato cheese, with ham (*Hormel* Micro Cup), 7.5 oz. . . 190
rice and beans, Cajun or Northern Italian (*Fantastic* Cup),
  2.3 oz. 240
rice and beans, Caribbean (*Fantastic* Cup), 2.1 oz. 230
rice and beans, curry, Bombay (*Fantastic* Cup), 2.3 oz. . . 260
rice and beans, Mexican (*Campbell's Soupsations*),
  1 pkg. 210
rice and beans, Szechuan (*Fantastic* Cup), 1.9 oz. 210
rice and beans, Tex-Mex (*Fantastic* Cup), 2.4 oz. 270
tomato rice Parmesano (*Fantastic* Cup), 1.9 oz. 200
tomato vegetable (*Campbell's Soupsations*), 1 pkg. 130
vegetable (*Campbell's* Soup/Recipe), 2 tbsp. 35
vegetable (*Lipton Recipe Secrets*), 2 tbsp. 30
vegetable, barley, hearty (*Fantastic* Cup), 1.5 oz. 150
Sour cream, see "Cream, sour"
Soy beverage:
(*EdenSoy/EdenSoy* Extra), 8 fl. oz. 130
(*Soy Moo* Fat Free), 8 fl. oz. 110
Soy sauce:
(*Kikkoman/Kikkoman* Light), 1 tbsp. 10
tamari (*Eden* Domestic), 1 tbsp. 15
shoyu (*Eden* Imported/Traditional), 1 tbsp. 15
Soybean:
green, boiled, drained, 1/2 cup 127
dried, raw (*Arrowhead Mills*), 1/4 cup 170
dried, dry-roasted, 1/2 cup 387
Soybean sprouts (*Jonathan's*), 1 cup, 3 oz. 100

Spaghetti, plain, see "Pasta"
Spaghetti dinner, and meatballs, frozen (*Swanson* Budget), 1 pkg. 300
Spaghetti dishes, mix, dry:
with meat sauce (*Kraft* Dinner), 5.5 oz. 330
mild or tangy (*Kraft* American Dinner), 2 oz. 200
Spaghetti entree, canned:
with meatballs (*Campbell's Superiore/Franco-American*), 1 cup 270
with meatballs (*Libby's Diner*), 7.75 oz. 190
tomato-cheese sauce (*Franco-American*), 1 cup 210
Spaghetti entree, frozen:
Bolognese (*Banquet*), 10.5 oz. 370
Bolognese (*Healthy Choice*), 10 oz. 260
marinara (*Marie Callender's*), 8 oz. 270
with meat sauce (*Lean Cuisine*), 11½ oz. 290
with meat sauce (*Marie Callender's*), 6.8 oz. 260
with meat sauce (*Morton*), 8.5 oz. 170
with meat sauce (*Stouffer's Lunch Express*), 9⅝ oz. . . . 320
with meat sauce (*Weight Watchers*), 10 oz. 290
with meatballs (*Lean Cuisine*), 9½ oz. 290
with meatballs (*Stouffer's*), 12⅝ oz. 420
Spaghetti sauce, see "Pasta sauce"
Spaghetti squash, baked or boiled, drained, ½ cup 23
Spinach:
fresh, raw, chopped, ½ cup 6
fresh, boiled, drained, ½ cup 21
canned (*Allens Popeye*), ½ cup 45
canned (*S&W*), ½ cup 30
frozen, leaf (*Seabrook*), 1 cup 20
frozen, in butter sauce, cut (*Green Giant*), ½ cup 40
Spinach dip (*Marie's*), 2 tbsp. 140
Spinach dishes, frozen:
creamed (*Green Giant*), ½ cup 80
creamed (*Seabrook*), ½ cup 120
creamed (*Stouffer's* Side Dish), ½ of 9-oz. pkg. 160
creamed (*Tabatchnick*), 7.5 oz. 60
feta pocket (*Amy's*), 1 piece 200
Indian (*Deep* Palak Paneer), 5 oz. 230

Spinach dishes ***(cont.)***
soufflé (*Stouffer's* Side Dish), 1/3 of 12-oz. pkg. 150
Spiny lobster, meat only, boiled or steamed, 4 oz. 138
Split peas, green, dry (*Arrowhead Mills*), 1/4 cup 170
Sprouts (see also specific bean and seed listings):
bean (*Frieda's*), 1 oz. 10
bean, canned (*La Choy*), 1 cup 10
hot and spicy (*Jonathan's*), 1 cup, 4 oz. 25
mixed (*Jonathan's* Gourmet), 1 cup, 3 oz. 20
mixed (*Shaw's* Premium), 2 oz. 9
mixed, lentil, adzuki, pea (*Jonathan's*), 3 oz. 100
Squab, fresh, raw, breast meat only, 4 oz. 161
Squash, canned (*Stokely*), 1/2 cup 50
Squid, meat only, raw, 4 oz. 104
Squid, canned, in juice (*Goya*), 1/4 cup 120
Steak sauce, 1 tbsp.:
(*A.1.*) 15
(*A.1.* Thick and Hearty) 25
(*Heinz 57*) 15
(*HP*) 15
(*Hunt's*) 10
(*Texas Best*) 15
and burger (*Try Me Bullfighter*) 15
garlic peppercorn or sweet-spicy (*Lea & Perrins*) 25
New Orleans style (*Trappey's Chef-Magic*) 10
Stir-fry entree, frozen, as packaged:
lo mein (*Green Giant Create A Meal!*), 2 1/3 cup 160
sweet and sour (*Green Giant Create A Meal!*), 2 3/4 cup . . 130
Szechuan or vegetable almond (*Green Giant Create A Meal!*), 2 3/4 cup 150
teriyaki (*Green Giant Create A Meal!*), 2 3/4 cup 100
teriyaki (*Lean Cuisine Lunch Express*), 9 oz. 260
Stir-fry sauce (see also "Marinade," and specific listings):
(*Ka-Me*), 1 tbsp. 10
(*Kikkoman*), 1 tbsp. 15
(*Lawry's*), 1 tbsp. 25
(*S&W* Oriental), 1 tbsp. 20
honey or regular (*Ken's Steak House*), 1 tbsp. 20

mandarin soy (*La Choy*), ½ cup 70
and rib, garlic (*Mi-Kee*), 1 tbsp. 30
spicy (*La Choy* Szechwan), ½ cup 85
sweet and sour, spicy (*La Choy*), ½ cup 140
teriyaki (*La Choy*), ½ cup 95

Strawberry:
fresh, ½ cup 23
frozen, unsweetened, ½ cup 26
frozen (*Stilwell*), ⅔ cup 50

Strawberry drink:
(*Capri Sun* Cooler), 6.75 fl. oz. 100
(*Farmer's Market*), 8 fl. oz. 120
nectar (*Kern's*), 8 fl. oz. 150

Strawberry drink blends, 8 fl. oz.:
banana or kiwi (*R.W. Knudsen/R.W. Knudsen* Cactus) . . 120
banana nectar (*Kern's*) 150
guava (*Santa Cruz*) 100
melon (*Veryfine* Shivering Chillers) 120
orange banana (*Tree Top*) 120

Strawberry juice, 8 fl. oz.:
(*Veryfine* Juice-Ups) 140
nectar (*R.W. Knudsen*) 120

Strawberry milk drink:
canned (*Sego*), 10 fl. oz. 240
canned, creme (*Carnation Instant Breakfast*), 10 fl. oz. . . 220
mix, powder, creme (*Carnation Instant Breakfast*), 1 pkt. 130

Strawberry syrup (*Knott's Berry Farm*), 2 tbsp. 120

Strawberry topping, 2 tbsp.:
(*Smucker's*) 100
Melba (*Dickinson's*) 90

Stroganoff gravy, with mushrooms (*Pepperidge Farm*), ¼ cup 30

Stroganoff seasoning mix (*Durkee Pouch*), ⅛ pkg. 10

Stuffing (see also "Stuffing mix"):
(*Arnold* Unspiced), 2 cups 250
Cajun rice (*Good Harvest*), ½ cup 130
corn bread or seasoned herb (*Pepperidge Farm*), ¾ cup 170
corn bread, honey pecan (*Pepperidge Farm*), ½ cup . . . 140
cube, bread, unseasoned (*Brownberry*), 2 cups 240

Stuffing *(cont.)*
garden and herb or sage and onion (*Pepperidge Farm*), ½ cup 150
Santa Fe (*Good Harvest*), ½ cup 110
sourdough, San Francisco (*Good Harvest*), ½ cup 110
vegetable, harvest, and almond (*Pepperidge Farm*), ½ cup 140
wild rice trio (*Good Harvest*), ½ cup 140

Stuffing mix:
(*Kellogg's Crouettes*), 1 cup 120
all varieties (*Rice-A-Roni*), 1 cup* 170
all varieties (*Stove Top*), ⅙ pkg. 110
all varieties (*Stove Top* Flexible Serve), 1 oz. 120
chicken flavor (*Stove Top* Microwave), ⅙ pkg. 130
corn bread, homestyle (*Stove Top* Microwave), ⅙ pkg. . . 120

Sturgeon, meat only:
baked, broiled, or microwaved, 4 oz. 153
smoked, 4 oz. 196

Subway, 1 serving, except as noted:
sandwiches:
bologna, jumbo 446
bologna, junior 270
ham, jumbo 259
ham, junior 208
roast beef, jumbo 348
roast beef, junior 232
Subway Seafood & Crab, jumbo 472
Subway Seafood & Crab, jumbo, with lite mayo 348
Subway Seafood & Crab, junior 279
Subway Seafood & Crab, junior, with lite mayo 238
tuna, jumbo 632
tuna, jumbo, with lite mayo 406
tuna, junior 332
tuna, junior, with lite mayo 257
turkey breast, jumbo 290
turkey breast, junior 218
submarines, cold, 6":
Classic Italian B.M.T. 434
ham 273

mixed cold cuts	347
roast beef	299
Subway Club	300
Subway Seafood & Crab	415
Subway Seafood & Crab with lite mayo	333
tuna	522
tuna with lite mayo	372
turkey breast	276
turkey breast and ham	275
Veggie Delite	223
submarines, hot, 6″:	
chicken breast, roasted	321
meatball	411
steak and cheese	363
Subway Melt	361
salads:	
bread bowl	290
chicken breast fillet, roasted	143
Subway Club	123
Subway Seafood & Crab	238
Subway Seafood & Crab with lite mayo	155
tuna	345
tuna with lite mayo	194
turkey breast	99
Veggie Delite	45
salad dressings, 1 tbsp.:	
French, creamy Italian, or Thousand Island	65
French, fat free	15
Italian, creamy	65
ranch	87
ranch, fat free	12
condiments and dressings:	
bacon, 2 slices	45
cheese, 2 triangles	41
mayonnaise dressing, 1 tsp.	37
mayonnaise dressing, lite, 1 tsp.	18
mustard, 2 tsp.	8
olive oil blend, 1 tsp.	45
vinegar, 1 tsp.	1

Subway*, condiments and dressings *(cont.)
cookies, 1.3-oz. piece:
chocolate, double with Brazil nut 200
chocolate, white with macadamias 174
chocolate chip, regular 161
chocolate chip, *M&M's* 162
chocolate chip, walnut 165
chocolate chip, white 166
chocolate chunk 160
oatmeal raisin 147
peanut butter 169
sugar 178
toffee crunch 153
Succotash, canned, whole kernel (*Stokely*), ½ cup 100
Sugar, beet or cane, 1 tbsp.:
brown 50
granulated 46
powdered or confectioner's, unsifted 31
Sugar, maple, 1 oz. 99
Sugar apple, 1 medium, 9.9 oz. 146
Summer sausage (*Old Smokehouse*), 1 oz. 110
Sunfish, meat only, baked, broiled, or microwaved, 4 oz. 129
Sunflower seed, 1 oz., except as noted:
dried, in shell (*Arrowhead Mills*), 1 cup, 1.3 oz. edible . . 180
dry-roasted, in shell (*Planters*), 3-oz. bag, 1.5 oz. edible 240
dry-roasted, kernels (*Planters*), ¼ cup, 1.1 oz. 190
honey-roasted, kernels (*Planters*), 1.7-oz. pkg. 280
oil-roasted, kernels (*Planters*), 1.7-oz. pkg. 290
Sunflower seed butter (*Roaster Fresh*), 1 oz. 160
Sunflower sprouts (*Jonathan's*), 1 cup, 3 oz. 45
Sweet potato, baked in skin, 1 medium 118
Sweet potato, canned, ½ cup, except as noted:
whole (*Royal Prince/Trappey's* Yam), 6 oz., 4 pieces . . . 200
halves (*Royal Prince*), 5.7 oz., 3 pieces 190
mashed (*Princella/Sugary Sam*), ⅔ cup 120
candied or orange-pineapple (*Royal Prince*) 210
candied (*S&W*) 170
Sweet potato, frozen:
baked, cubed, ½ cup 88

candied (*Mrs. Paul's*), 5 fl. oz. 300
candied (*Ore-Ida*), 5 pieces 170
candied, with apples (*Mrs. Paul's* Sweets'n Apples), 1 cup 270
Sweet potato chips, regular or cinnamon spice (*Terra* Chips), 1 oz. 140
Sweet and sour dinner mix (*La Choy*), 1/4 pkg. 90
Sweet and sour drink mixer (*Holland House*), 4 fl. oz. . . 100
Sweet and sour sauce:
(*Kikkoman*), 2 tbsp. 35
(*Woody's*), 2 tbsp. 70
chicken (*Gold's Dip'n Joy*), 1 tbsp. 30
duck sauce (*Ka-Me*), 2 tbsp. 80
duck sauce, all varieties (*Gold's*), 2 tbsp. 60
or duck sauce (*La Choy*), 2 tbsp. 60
Sweetbreads, see "Pancreas" and "Thymus"
Swiss chard, boiled, drained, chopped, 1/2 cup 18
Swiss steak gravy mix (*Durkee*), 1/4 cup* 15
Swordfish, fresh, meat only, baked, broiled, or microwaved, 4 oz. 176
Swordfish, frozen, steaks (*Peter Pan*), 4 oz. 160
Syrup, see specific listings
Szechuan sauce (see also "Stir-fry sauce"):
(*Ka-Me*), 1 tbsp. 20
cooking (*Kylin* Chili & Tomato), 1/4 cup 50

T

FOOD AND MEASURE	CALORIES
Tabouli (*Frieda's*), ½ cup	152
Tabouli mix:	
(*Fantastic*), ¼ cup	120
(*Near East*), ⅔ cup*	120
Taco Bell, 1 serving:	
burritos:	
bean	391
beef	432
big beef *Burrito Supreme*	525
Burrito Supreme	443
chicken	345
chicken *Burrito Supreme*	520
chili cheese	391
combo	412
7 layer	485
steak *Burrito Supreme*	500
tacos and tostados:	
soft taco, regular or chicken	223
soft taco, steak	217
soft taco, *Taco Supreme*	268
taco	180
Taco Supreme	225
tostada	242
sauces, sides, and specialty items:	
beef *MexiMelt*	262
cinnamon twists	139
guacamole	36
Mexican pizza	574
nachos	345
nachos *BellGrande*	633
nachos supreme	364
nacho cheese sauce	51
pintos 'n cheese	190

ranch dressing 136
salsa 27
seasoned rice 110
taco salad 838
Taco entree, frozen, mini (*Swanson Fun Feast*), 1 pkg. 380
Taco mix, dinner (*Lawry's*), 1/5 pkg. 150
Taco sauce:
(*Hunt's Manwich*), 1/4 cup 30
(*Lawry's* Chunky), 2 tbsp. 10
red (*La Victoria*), 1 tbsp. 5
Taco seasoning mix:
(*Lawry's*), 1 tbsp. 25
regular or mild (*Durkee* Pouch), 1/8 pkg. 15
salad (*Durkee* Pouch), 1/6 pkg. 20
Taco shell (see also "Tortilla"):
(*Lawry's*), 2 shells 120
(*Rosarita*), 3 shells 155
tostada (*Lawry's*), 2 shells 110
tostada (*Rosarita*), 2 shells 125
white corn (*Chi-Chi's*), 2 shells 170
Tagliatelle, spinach, refrigerated (*Contadina*), 1 1/4 cup . . 270
Tahini (*Joyva*), 2 tbsp. 200
Tahini sauce mix (*Casbah*), 1 oz. 160
Tamale, canned:
(*Gebhardt*), 2 pieces 270
(*Gebhardt* Jumbo), 2 pieces 330
(*Just Rite*), 3 pieces 255
(*Old El Paso*), 3 pieces 330
(*Van Camp's*), 2 pieces 210
beef (*Hormel*), 7.5-oz. can 290
beef, hot-spicy or regular (*Hormel*), 3 pieces, 7.5 oz. . . . 280
beef, jumbo (*Hormel*), 2 pieces, 7 oz. 270
chicken (*Hormel*), 3 pieces, 7.5 oz. 210
Tamale pie, Mexican, frozen (*Amy's*), 8 oz. 220
Tamarind, pulp (*Frieda's* Tamarindo), 3.5 oz. 239
Tandoori paste, mild (*Patak's*), 2 tbsp. 30
Tangerine:
fresh, 1 medium, 2 3/8" diameter 37
canned, in juice (*S&W* Natural Style Mandarin), 2/3 cup . . . 70

Tangerine ***(cont.)***
canned, in light syrup (*Del Monte*), ½ cup 80
canned, in light syrup (*S&W* Mandarin), ⅔ cup 100
Tangerine juice:
fresh, 6 fl. oz. 80
frozen* (*Minute Maid* Beverage), 8 fl. oz. 120
blend (*Dole* Mandarin), 8 fl. oz. 140
Tapioca, dry (*Minute*), 1½ tsp. 20
Tapioca pudding, see "Pudding"
Taro, cooked (*Frieda's*), 5 oz. 150
Taro chips, spiced (*Terra* Chips), 1 oz. 130
Taro root, cooked (*Frieda's*), 5 oz. 150
Tartar sauce (*Hellmann's/Best Foods*), 2 tbsp. 140
TCBY:
soft-serve yogurt, all flavors, ½ cup:
  regular 130
  nonfat 110
  nonfat, no sugar 80
sorbet, all flavors, ½ cup 100
premium nonfat yogurt, ½ cup:
  apple pie à la mode 120
  banana split 110
  cappuccino 120
  chocolate, brown/white or chewy sundae 120
  peach cobbler 110
  raspberry or strawberry cheesecake 120
  vanilla caramel custard 120
Yog·A·Bar, 1 bar:
  orange or raspberry swirl 80
  vanilla, chocolate dipped 120
  vanilla, with toasted almonds or with *Heath* toffee . . . 190
Tea, iced, 8 fl. oz., except as noted:
(*Schweppes*) 90
(*Snapple*) 70
all fruit flavors (*Apple & Eve*) 100
all fruit flavors (*Lipton* Chilled) 80
all fruit flavors, herbal (*R.W. Knudsen* Coolers) 90
lemon, peach, raspberry, or strawberry (*Snapple*) 100
lemon (*Veryfine* Chillers) 90

mango or passion fruit (*Snapple*) 110
mint (*Snapple*) 120
peach or raspberry (*Snapple*), 11.5 fl. oz. 150
peach-kiwi or plain (*Veryfine* Chillers) 80
raspberry (*Veryfine* Chillers) 100
Tempeh, 1 oz. 56
Teriyaki sauce, 1 tbsp.:
(*House of Tsang Korean Teriyaki*) 30
(*La Choy/La Choy* Lite) 20
baste and glaze (*Kikkoman*) 50
baste and glaze, honey and pineapple (*Kikkoman*) 80
hot (*La Choy* Chun King) 20
marinade (*Lawry's*) 20
marinade and sauce (*Kikkoman/Kikkoman* Light) 15
Teriyaki seasoning mix, beef (*Durkee* Pouch), 1/5 pkg., 1 tbsp. 30
Thai sauce (*World Harbors* Nong Khai), 1 tbsp. 20
Thymus:
beef, braised, 4 oz. 362
veal, braised, 4 oz. 197
Tilefish, meat only, baked, broiled, or microwaved, 4 oz. 167
Tofu, fresh:
extra firm (*Nasoya*), 1/5 of 1-lb. block 90
firm (*Nasoya*), 1/5 of 1-lb. block 80
silken (*Nasoya*), 1/5 of 1-lb. block 50
soft (*Nasoya*), 1/6 of 1-lb. block 60
flavored, 5-spice or French country (*Nasoya*), 1/4 block, 3 oz. 70
Tofu dishes, mix:
burger (*Fantastic* Classics), 1/8 cup dry 70
chow mein, mandarin (*Fantastic* Classics), 1 cup with tofu* 330
shells 'n curry (*Fantastic* Classics), 1 cup with tofu* . . . 440
Stroganoff, creamy (*Fantastic* Classics), 1 cup with tofu* 430
Tofu seasoning mix, 1/4 pkg.:
all flavors, except stir fry (*Tofu-Mate*) 15
breakfast scramble (*Fantastic* Classics) 60
stir fry, Mandarin (*Tofu-Mate*) 30
stir fry, Szechuan (*Tofu-Mate*) 25

Tom collins mixer, bottled (*Holland House*), 3 fl. oz. . . . 160
Tomatillo:
fresh, 1 medium, 1⅝" diam. or ¼ cup chopped 11
canned (*La Victoria* Entero), 5 pieces 40
canned, crushed (*La Victoria*), 4.5 oz. 45
Tomato, fresh, ripe (see also "Tomato, canned" and "Tomato, dried or sun-dried"):
raw, 2⅗"-diam. tomato 26
raw, chopped, ½ cup 19
boiled, ½ cup 32
Tomato, canned (see also "Tomato sauce, canned"), ½ cup, except as noted:
(*Hunt's*) 30
aspic (*S&W*) 50
crushed (*Hunt's*) 30
crushed (*S&W*), ¼ cup 20
cut (*Hunt's* Choice Cut) 20
cut, in juice (*S&W* Ready-Cut/Ready-Cut Italian) 25
cut, in puree (*S&W* Ready-Cut) 30
diced, with roasted garlic or Italian herbs (*Hunt's* Choice Cut) 25
with green chilies, diced (*Chi-Chi's*), ¼ cup 20
stewed (*Hunt's*) 35
stewed, all varieties, except Italian (*Del Monte*) 35
stewed, Italian (*Del Monte*) 30
stewed, Italian (*S&W*) 35
whole, regular or pear (*Hunt's*), 2 pieces 20
whole, Italian pear with basil or peeled (*S&W*) 25
Tomato, dried or sun-dried:
½ cup, approx. 15 pieces 70
(*Frieda's* No Salt), 1 oz. 86
bits (*Sonoma*), 2–3 tsp. 15
flakes (*Christopher Ranch*), 3 tbsp. 80
halves (*Sonoma*), 2–3 pieces 15
in oil, drained (*Sonoma* Spice Medley), 1 tbsp. 50
pasta toss (*Sonoma*), ½ cup 70
seasoning (*Sonoma* Season It), 2–3 tsp. 20
Tomato, green, 2⅗"-diam. tomato 30
Tomato, pickled (*Claussen*), 1 oz. 5

Tomato dip, sun-dried (*Marie's*), 2 tbsp. 140
Tomato juice, 8 fl. oz.:
(*Campbell's/Campbell's* Enhanced Flavor Low Sodium) . . . 50
(*Hunt's/Hunt's* No Salt) 35
(*Sacramento*) 35
(*S&W*) 40
Tomato paste, 2 tbsp.:
(*Contadina*) 30
(*S&W*) 30
plain or flavored (*Hunt's*) 30
Italian (*Contadina*) 40
Tomato puree, 1/4 cup:
(*Contadina*) 20
(*Hunt's*) 25
Tomato sauce, canned, 1/4 cup, except as noted:
(*Contadina/Contadina* Thick & Zesty) 20
(*Hunt's/Hunt's* No Salt) 15
(*S&W*) 20
chili, chunky (*Hunt's Ready Sauce*) 20
chunky (*Hunt's Ready Sauce*) 15
chunky (*Hunt's Ready Sauce* Special) 20
garden, regular or mild Mexican (*S&W/S&W* Original) . . . 20
garden, Italian herb (*S&W*), 1/2 cup 35
garlic (*Hunt's Ready Sauce*) 30
garlic and herb or chunky Italian (*Hunt's Ready Sauce*) . 25
herb or Italian (*Hunt's*) 30
herb, country (*Hunt's Ready Sauce*) 35
herb and garlic (*S&W* Cooking Sauce), 1 tbsp. 15
meat loaf, Mexican, or salsa (*Hunt's Ready Sauce*) 20
Tomato tapenade, dried (*Sonoma*), 1 tbsp. 70
Tomato-chile cocktail (*Snap-E-Tom*), 6 fl. oz. 40
Tongue, beef, braised, 4 oz. 321
Tongue lunch meat, beef, corned (*Hebrew National*),
2 oz. 120
Tortellini, frozen or refrigerated:
cheese, three (*Contadina*), 3/4 cup 260
cheese, three, spinach (*Contadina*), 3/4 cup 260
mushroom (*Contadina*), 1 cup 310
spinach (*Putney*), 1 cup 290

Tortellini entree, canned, 1 cup:
cheese (*Chef Boyardee*) 230
cheese (*Franco-American*) 240
meat (*Chef Boyardee*) 260
meat (*Franco-American*) 260
meat, ground beef (*Chef Boyardee* Bowl), 7.5 oz. 220

Tortilla:
corn, yellow (*Tyson*), 3 pieces 140
flour (*Mesa*), 6" piece 80
flour (*Tyson*), 1.9 oz. 170
flour, heat pressed (*Tyson*), 2 pieces 180

Tortilla chips, see "Corn chips, puffs, and similar snacks"

Trail mix:
(*Sonoma*), 1/4 cup 160
California (*Dole*), 1.2 oz. 130
Hawaiian (*Dole*), 1.2 oz. 150
Sierra (*Del Monte*), 1 oz. 120

Trout (see also "Sea trout"), meat only:
mixed species, baked, broiled, or microwaved, 4 oz. . . . 215
rainbow, farmed, baked, broiled, or microwaved, 4 oz. . . 192
rainbow, wild, baked, broiled, or microwaved, 4 oz. 170
smoked, peppered, rainbow (*Spence & Co.*), 2 oz. 100

Tuna, meat only, 4 oz.:
bluefin, baked, broiled, or microwaved 209
skipjack, baked, broiled, or microwaved 150
yellowfin, baked, broiled, or microwaved 158

Tuna, canned, drained, 2 oz.:
chunk light, in oil (*Bumble Bee*) 110
chunk light, in oil (*Chicken of the Sea*) 110
chunk light, in oil (*S&W*) 110
chunk light, in oil (*Star-Kist*) 110
chunk light, in water (*Bumble Bee*) 60
chunk light, in water (*S&W*) 70
chunk white, in water (*Bumble Bee* Low Salt) 70
solid light, in water (*Star-Kist/Star-Kist* Prime Catch) 60
solid white, in oil (*Bumble Bee*) 90
solid white, in oil (*Chicken of the Sea*) 90
solid white, in oil (*S&W*) 80

solid white, in oil (*Star-Kist*) 90
solid white, albacore, in water (*Bumble Bee*) 70
Tuna, frozen, yellowtail (*Peter Pan*), 4 oz. 110
"Tuna," vegetarian, frozen (*Worthington Tuno*), ½ cup
drained 80
Tuna entree, frozen:
noodle casserole (*Stouffer's*), 10 oz. 320
noodle casserole (*Swanson*), 1 pkg. 320
Tuna entree mix*:
broccoli, creamy (*Tuna Helper*), ⅔ cup 190
cheddar, garden (*Tuna Helper*), ⅔ cup 190
pasta, cheesy (*Tuna Helper*), ¾ cup 170
pasta, creamy (*Tuna Helper*), ¾ cup 190
pot pie (*Tuna Helper*), ½ cup 340
Tuna salad spread (*Libby's Spreadables*), ⅓ cup 130
Turbot, European, meat only, baked, broiled, or
microwaved, 4 oz. 138
Turkey, fresh, roasted, 4 oz., except as noted:
meat with skin 236
meat only 193
meat only, diced, 1 cup 238
dark meat, with skin 251
dark meat, meat only 212
dark meat, meat only, diced, 1 cup 262
light meat, with skin 223
light meat, meat only 178
light meat, meat only, diced, 1 cup 219
breast, meat with skin, ½ breast, 1.9 lb. (4.2 lbs. raw
with bone) 1637
leg, meat with skin, 1 leg, 1.2 lb. (1.5 lbs. raw with
bone) 1133
wing, meat with skin, 1 wing, 6.6 oz. (9.9 oz. raw with
bone) 426
Turkey, canned, chunk, 2 oz. or ¼ cup:
(*Hormel*) 70
(*Swanson* Premium) 100
white (*Hormel*) 60
white (*Swanson* Premium) 90

Turkey, frozen or refrigerated, 3 oz., except as noted:
whole, cooked, dark meat (*Perdue*) 200
whole, cooked, white meat (*Perdue*) 170
breast, cooked (*Perdue* Whole/Half) 170
breast, cooked, boneless, fillets or tenderloins (*Perdue*) 110
breast, cooked, cutlets, thin sliced (*Perdue*), 2.5 oz. 90
breast, honey roasted or smoked (*Louis Rich*),
2.8-oz. slice 80
breast, oven roasted (*Louis Rich*), 2.8-oz. slice 70
breast, smoked (*Perdue*) 150
maple glazed (*Boar's Head Honey Coat*) 100
steak, cubed, raw (*Perdue*), 4 oz. 110
thigh, cooked (*Perdue*) 180
wing, roasted (*Perdue*), 3-oz. wing 180
Turkey, ground (see also "Turkey patty"):
raw (*Louis Rich*), 4 oz. 190
raw, breast meat (*Perdue*), 4 oz. 120
raw, regular or burger (*Perdue*), 4 oz. 160
cooked, breast meat (*Perdue*), 3 oz. 110
cooked, regular or burger (*Perdue*), 3 oz. 170
"Turkey," vegetarian:
canned (*Worthington* Turkee), 3 slices 130
frozen, smoked, sliced (*Worthington*), 3 slices 140
Turkey bacon (*Louis Rich*), .5-oz. slice 30
Turkey bologna:
(*Louis Rich*), 1-oz. slice 50
(*Norbest*), 2 oz. 130
Turkey chili, see "Chili, canned"
Turkey dinner, frozen:
breast (*Healthy Choice*), 10.5 oz. 280
breast meat, with pasta (*Swanson*), 1 pkg. 270
mostly white meat (*Swanson*), 1 pkg. 300
mostly white meat (*Swanson Hungry Man*), 1 pkg. 510
and gravy, with dressing (*Banquet*), 18.8 oz. 560
with gravy, dressing (*Marie Callender's*), 14 oz. 530
Turkey entree, canned:
gravy and dressing (*Dinty Moore American Classics*),
10-oz. bowl 290
gravy and dressing (*Libby's Diner*), 7 oz. 180

stew (*Dinty Moore*), 1 cup 150
Turkey entree, frozen:
(*Lean Cuisine* Homestyle), 9$\frac{3}{8}$ oz. 230
breast, stuffed (*Weight Watchers*), 9 oz. 230
fettuccine alla crema (*Healthy Choice*), 12.5 oz. 350
glazed (*Lean Cuisine* Cafe Classics), 9 oz. 250
and gravy, with dressing (*Banquet* Homestyle), 9.25 oz. 270
and gravy, with dressing (*Swanson*), 1 pkg. 230
gravy and (*Banquet* Toppers), 5-oz. bag 90
gravy and, with dressing (*Morton*), 9 oz. 230
pie (*Banquet*), 7 oz. 370
pie (*Empire* Kosher), 6.6 oz. 470
pie (*Lean Cuisine*), 9$\frac{1}{2}$ oz. 300
pie (*Marie Callender's*), 10 oz. 710
pie (*Stouffer's*), 10 oz. 530
pie (*Swanson*), 1 pkg. 440
pie (*Swanson Hungry Man*), 1 pkg. 650
pie (*Tyson*), 9 oz. 550
roast (*Healthy Choice* Country Inn), 10 oz. 250
roast, breast, and stuffing (*Lean Cuisine*), 9$\frac{3}{4}$ oz. 290
roast, with mushrooms (*Healthy Choice* Country), 8.5 oz. 220
roast, and stuffing (*Stouffer's* Homestyle), 7$\frac{7}{8}$ oz. 280
tetrazzini (*Stouffer's*), 10 oz. 360
Turkey frankfurter, 1 link:
(*Empire* Kosher), 2 oz. 90
and beef (*Oscar Mayer* Hot Dogs), 1.75 oz. 40
and chicken (*Louis Rich* $\frac{8}{12}$ oz.), 1.5 oz. 80
and chicken (*Louis Rich Bun-Length*), 2 oz. 110
Turkey gravy, $\frac{1}{4}$ cup:
roasted (*Heinz* Home Style) 25
seasoned, with turkey (*Pepperidge Farm*) 30
mix*, roasted (*Knorr*) 25
Turkey ham, 2 oz., except as noted:
(*Healthy Deli*) 70
canned (*Hormel*) 70
chopped (*Louis Rich*), 1-oz. slice 40
honey cured or regular (*Louis Rich*), 3 slices, 2.2 oz. . . 70
Turkey ham, canned (*Hormel*), 2 oz. 70
Turkey hash, roast, canned (*Mary Kitchen*), 1 cup 210

Turkey lunch meat (see also "Turkey ham," etc.), breast:
(*Hormel* Deli Premium), 2 oz. .50
all varieties, except oven roasted Italian style (*Healthy Deli*), 2 oz. 60
honey roasted or regular (*Hormel Light & Lean* 97), 2 oz. 50
lemon garlic (*Hebrew National*), 5 thin slices, 1.8 oz. 50
maple honey or hickory smoked (*Boar's Head*), 2 oz. 70
oven roasted (*Boar's Head* Golden/Golden Skinless), 2 oz. 60
oven roasted (*Hebrew National*), 5 thin slices, 1.8 oz. 50
oven roasted (*Oscar Mayer*), 1-oz. slice 25
oven roasted, Italian style (*Healthy Deli*), 2 oz. 70
oven roasted, white (*Oscar Mayer Deli-Thin*), 4 slices, 1.8 oz. 50
roast (*Oscar Mayer Deli-Thin*), 4 slices, 1.8 oz. 50
smoked (*Boar's Head Cracked Pepper Mill*), 2 oz. 60
smoked (*Hebrew National*), 5 thin slices, 1.8 oz. 60
smoked (*Hebrew National* Hickory), 2 oz. 60
smoked (*Hormel* Mesquite), 2 oz. 60
smoked, hickory (*Boar's Head* Hickory), 2 oz. 70
smoked, honey roasted (*Oscar Mayer Deli-Thin*), 4 slices, 1.8 oz. 60
Turkey nuggets, breaded (*Louis Rich*), 4 pieces, 3.25 oz. 260
Turkey pastrami, 2 oz.:
(*Boar's Head*) 60
(*Healthy Deli*) 70
(*Hebrew National*) 60
Turkey patty, breaded:
(*Empire* Kosher), 3.1-oz. patty 200
(*Louis Rich*), 3-oz. patty 220
Turkey salad spread (*Libby's Spreadables*), ⅓ cup 150
Turkey salami:
(*Empire* Kosher), 3 slices, 1.8 oz. 70
(*Louis Rich*), 2 oz. 120
cotto (*Louis Rich*), 1-oz. slice 40
Turkey sandwich, frozen, 1 piece:
with broccoli (*Mrs. Paterson's Aussie Pie*) 470
with broccoli and cheese (*Lean Pockets*) 260

with broccoli and cheese or ham with cheddar (*Hot Pockets*) 320

Turkey sausage:

(*Shady Brook Farms* Old World), 4 oz. raw 190

breakfast, cooked (*Perdue*), 2 links 100

Italian, hot or sweet, raw (*Shady Brook Farms*), 4 oz. . . 170

Italian, hot or sweet, raw or cooked (*Perdue*), 1 link . . . 110

Turkey sticks, breaded (*Louis Rich*), 3 sticks, 3 oz. 230

Turnip:

fresh or stored, boiled, drained, cubed, ½ cup 14

frozen, boiled, drained, 4 oz. 26

Turnip greens, ½ cup:

fresh, raw, chopped 7

fresh, boiled, drained, chopped 15

canned (*Allens/Sunshine*) 25

canned, chopped, with diced turnip (*Allens/Sunshine*) . . . 30

frozen, with diced turnips (*Seabrook*) 30

Turnover, frozen or refrigerated, 1 piece, except as noted:

apple (*Pillsbury*), 2 pieces 350

apple, iced (*Pepperidge Farm*) 360

apple, cherry, or strawberry, mini (*Pepperidge Farm*) . . . 140

apple or raspberry (*Pepperidge Farm*) 330

blueberry (*Pepperidge Farm*) 340

cherry (*Pepperidge Farm*) 320

cherry (*Pillsbury*), 2 pieces 360

cherry, iced (*Pepperidge Farm*) 340

peach (*Pepperidge Farm*) 340

peach cobbler, mini (*Pepperidge Farm*) 160

raspberry, iced (*Pepperidge Farm*) 360

Tzatziki (*Western Creamy*), 2 tbsp. 60

V

FOOD AND MEASURE	CALORIES
Vanilla flavor drink:	
canned (*Sego*), 10 fl. oz.	240
canned, creme (*Sweet Success*), 10 fl. oz.	200
mix, creamy (*Sweet Success*), 1 pkt.	90
mix, French (*Carnation Instant Breakfast*), 1 pkt.	130
Veal, meat only, 4 oz.:	
cubed, lean only, braised or stewed	213
ground, broiled	195
leg, roasted, lean with fat	181
leg, roasted, lean only	170
loin, roasted, lean with fat	246
loin, roasted, lean only	198
rib, roasted, lean with fat	259
rib, roasted, lean only	201
shoulder, arm, braised, lean with fat	268
shoulder, arm, braised, lean only	228
shoulder, arm, roasted, lean with fat	208
shoulder, arm, roasted, lean only	186
shoulder, blade, braised, lean with fat	255
shoulder, blade, braised, lean only	224
shoulder, blade, roasted, lean with fat	211
shoulder, blade, roasted, lean only	194
sirloin, roasted, lean with fat	229
sirloin, roasted, lean only	191
"Veal," vegetarian, frozen (*Worthington Veelets*), 1 patty	180
Veal dinner, parmigiana, frozen:	
(*Swanson*), 1 pkg.	400
(*Swanson Hungry Man*), 1 pkg.	640
Veal entree, parmigiana, frozen:	
(*Banquet*), 9 oz.	320
(*Morton*), 8.75 oz.	280
(*Swanson*), 1 pkg.	310

patties (*Banquet* Family), 1 patty 230
with spaghetti (*Stouffer's* Homestyle), 11⅞ oz. 420
Vegetable antipasto, in jars (*Paesana*), 3¾ oz. 260
Vegetable burger, see " 'Hamburger,' vegetarian"
Vegetable chips (*Eden*), 50 chips, 1.1 oz. 130
Vegetable dinner, frozen:
(*Amy's* Country), 11 oz. 380
loaf (*Amy's*), 10 oz. 260
Vegetable dishes, frozen (see also specific listings):
pocket, see "Vegetable pocket"
samosa (*Deep* Indian Cuisine), 2 pieces 130
Vegetable entree, canned or in jars:
Chinese, mixed (*La Choy*), ⅔ cup 15
chop suey (*La Choy*), ⅔ cup 15
curry (*Patak's*), ½ cup 180
Vegetable entree, frozen:
country, and beef (*Lean Cuisine*), 9 oz. 220
pilaf, Indian (*Deep*), 1 cup 230
pie (*Amy's*), 7.5 oz. 360
pie (*Amy's* Nondairy), 7.5 oz. 320
pie, with cheese (*Banquet*), 7 oz. 390
pie, with beef (*Morton*), 7 oz. 310
pie, with chicken (*Morton*), 7 oz. 320
pie, with turkey (*Morton*), 7 oz. 300
shepherd's pie, nondairy (*Amy's*), 8 oz. 160
Vegetable entree mix, stew (*Knorr* Cup), 1 pkg. 160
Vegetable juice, 8 fl. oz.:
all varieties (*R.W. Knudsen Very Veggie*) 50
low sodium or lightly tangy (*V-8*) 60
picante, regular or spicy hot (*V-8*) 50
Vegetable pocket (see also specific listings), frozen,
1 piece:
Bar-B-Q (*Ken & Robert's Veggie Pockets*) 290
Greek, Oriental, or Santa Fe (*Ken & Robert's Veggie Pockets*) 250
Indian (*Ken & Robert's Veggie Pockets*) 260
pot pie (*Amy's*) 230
pot pie (*Ken & Robert's Veggie Pockets*) 250
Tex-Mex (*Ken & Robert's Veggie Pockets*) 280

Vegetables, mixed, fresh, 3 oz.:
California, garden, or Oriental style (*Dole*) 30
Italian style (*Dole*) 25
New England (*Dole*) 50
Vegetables, mixed, canned, ½ cup, except as noted:
(*S&W*) 35
(*Stokely/Stokely* No Salt) 35
Chinese (*La Choy*), ⅔ cup 10
chop suey (*La Choy*) 15
and sauce (*House of Tsang* Cantonese Classic/Szechuan) . 70
and sauce, sweet and sour (*House of Tsang* Hong King) 160
and sauce, teriyaki (*House of Tsang* Tokyo) 100
stew (*Stokely*) 45
Vegetables, mixed, frozen:
(*Green Giant*), ¾ cup 50
(*Green Giant Harvest Fresh*), ⅔ cup 50
butter sauce (*Green Giant*), ¾ cup 70
California or Seattle (*Green Giant*), ¾ cup 25
English, cheddar (*Green Giant* International), 4 oz. 120
French, garlic-Dijon (*Green Giant* International), 4 oz. 60
Heartland (*Green Giant*), 1 cup 30
Italian Parmesan (*Green Giant* International), 4 oz. 70
Japanese, teriyaki (*Green Giant* International), 4 oz. 50
Manhattan (*Green Giant*), 1 cup 25
New England (*Green Giant*), ⅔ cup 70
Normandy, mushroom (*Green Giant* International), 4 oz. . 80
San Francisco (*Green Giant*), ¾ cup 30
Santa Fe (*Green Giant*), ¾ cup 60
stew (*Ore-Ida*), ⅔ cup 50
stir-fry, see "Stir-fry entree"
Western (*Green Giant*), ¾ cup 50
Vegetables, mixed, pickled (*Zorba* Gardiniera), ½ cup . 20
Vegetarian entree (see also "Vegetable entree" and specific listings):
canned (*Loma Linda Swiss Stake*), 1 piece 120
canned (*Worthington Numete*), ⅜" slice 130
canned (*Worthington Protose*), ⅜" slice 130
canned, choplet (*Worthington*), 2 slices 90
canned, cutlet (*Worthington*), 1 slice 70

canned, cutlet, multigrain (*Worthington* 20 oz.), 2 slices 100
canned, cutlet, multigrain (*Worthington* 50 oz.), 1 slice . . . 80
canned, cuts, dinner (*Loma Linda*), 2 slices 90
frozen (*Worthington FriPats*), 1 patty 130
frozen (*Worthington Stakelets*), 1 piece 140
frozen, entree, dinner (*Natural Touch*), 3-oz. patty 220
frozen, croquettes (*Worthington* Golden), 4 pieces 210
frozen, roast, dinner (*Worthington*), 3/4" slice 180
Venison, meat only, roasted, 4 oz. 179
Vienna sausage, canned:
(*Hormel*), 2 oz. 140
(*Libby's/Libby's* BBQ), 3 links 130
chicken (*Hormel*), 2 oz. 110
chicken (*Libby's*), 3 links 100
Vine spinach, raw, untrimmed, 1 lb. 86
Vinegar, 1 tbsp.:
all varieties (*S&W*) 0
balsamic (*Pastorelli Italian Chef*) 5
red wine (*Pastorelli Italian Chef*) 2
Vodka sour mixer, instant (*Bar-Tenders*), 2 pouches,
1.1 oz. 110

W

FOOD AND MEASURE	CALORIES
Waffle, frozen, 2 pieces:	
(*Downyflake* Butter & Syrup)	150
(*Downyflake* Crisp & Healthy/Homestyle Jumbo)	170
(*Downyflake* Hot 'n Buttery)	180
(*Eggo* Homestyle)	220
(*Eggo Nutri-Grain*)	190
(*Kellogg's Special K*)	140
apple cinnamon, blueberry, buttermilk, or strawberry (*Eggo*)	220
blueberry (*Aunt Jemima*)	190
buttermilk, oatmeal, or whole grain (*Aunt Jemima*)	170
cinnamon (*Aunt Jemima*)	180
nut and honey (*Eggo*)	240
Waffle mix, see "Pancake mix"	
Walnut, dried:	
black (*Planters*), 2-oz. pkg.	340
black, chopped, 1 cup	759
English or Persian, shelled, 1 oz.	182
halves (*Planters*), 1/3 cup, 1.2 oz.	220
halves (*Planters Gold Measure*), 2-oz. pkg.	380
pieces (*Planters*), 1/4 cup, 1 oz.	190
Walnut topping, in syrup (*Smucker's*), 2 tbsp.	190
Water chestnuts, canned, Chinese:	
(*La Choy*), 2 pieces or 2 tbsp. slices	10
sliced (*Sun Luck*), 1/4 cup	15
Watercress, chopped, 1/2 cup	2
Watermelon:	
1 slice, 10″ diameter × 1″ thick	152
diced, 1/2 cup	25
seedless (*Frieda's*), 1 oz.	7
Watermelon drink (*R.W. Knudsen* Cooler), 8 fl. oz.	120
Watermelon juice (*After the Fall*), 8 fl. oz.	90

Wax beans:
fresh, see "Green beans"
canned, cut (*S&W*), ½ cup 20
canned, cut (*Stokely/Stokely* No Salt), ½ cup 20
frozen, 1″ pieces (*Seabrook*), ⅔ cup 25
Wax gourd, boiled, drained, cubed, ½ cup 11
Welsh rarebit, frozen (*Stouffer's*), 2.2 oz. 120
Wendy's, 1 serving:
sandwiches:
  bacon cheeseburger, Jr. 410
  Big Bacon Classic 610
  cheeseburger, Jr., or Kid's Meal 320
  cheeseburger deluxe, Jr. 360
  chicken, grilled 290
  chicken, breaded or spicy 440
  chicken club 500
  hamburger, single, plain 360
  hamburger, single, with everything 420
  hamburger, Jr., or Kid's Meal 270
chicken nuggets, 5 pieces 230
nuggets sauce, 1 oz.:
  barbecue 50
  honey 45
  honey mustard 130
  spicy buffalo wing 30
  sweet and sour 50
chili, large, 12 oz. 310
chili, small, 8 oz. 210
potatoes:
  baked, plain 310
  baked, bacon and cheese 540
  baked, broccoli and cheese 470
  baked, cheese 570
  baked, chili and cheese 620
  baked, sour cream with chive 380
  fries, small 260
  fries, medium 380
  fries, Biggie 460

Wendy's*, potatoes *(cont.)

salads-to-go, fresh, without dressing:

deluxe garden or side Caesar	110
grilled chicken	200
side salad	60
taco salad	510
soft bread stick	130

dressing, 2 tbsp.:

blue cheese	170
French	120
French, fat free	30
French, sweet red	130
Italian, reduced fat and calorie	40
Italian Caesar	150
ranch, *Hidden Valley*	90
ranch, *Hidden Valley,* reduced fat and calorie	60
Thousand Island	130

Garden Spot salad bar:

applesauce, 2 tbsp.	30
bacon bits, 2 tbsp.	45
banana/strawberry glaze, 1/4 cup	30
broccoli or cauliflower, 1/4 cup	0
cantaloupe, 1 slice	15
carrots, 1/4 cup	5
cheese, shredded, 2 tbsp.	50
chicken salad, 2 tbsp.	70
chow mein noodles, 1/4 cup	35
coleslaw, 2 tbsp.	45
cottage cheese, 2 tbsp.	30
croutons, 2 tbsp.	30
cucumbers or green pepper, 2 slices	0
eggs, hard-cooked, 2 tbsp.	40
green peas, 2 tbsp.	15
honeydew or watermelon, 1 slice or wedge	20
lettuce, 1 cup	10
mushrooms, 1/2 cup	0
orange, 2 slices	15
Parmesan blend, grated, 2 tbsp.	70
pasta salad, 2 tbsp.	25

peaches, 1 slice 15
pepperoni, 6 slices 30
pineapple chunks, 4 pieces 20
potato salad, 2 tbsp. 80
pudding, 1/4 cup 70
red onion, 3 rings 0
seafood salad, 1/4 cup 70
sesame bread stick, 1 piece 15
strawberries, 1 piece 10
sunflower seeds and raisins, 2 tbsp. 80
tomato wedges, 1 piece 5
turkey ham, diced, 2 tbsp. 50
desserts:
chocolate chip cookie 270
Frosty, small 340
Frosty, medium 460
Frosty, large 570
Wheat, whole grain, hard red, winter (*Arrowhead Mills*),
1/4 cup 160
Wheat bran (see also "Cereal"), 1/4 cup:
(*Arrowhead Mills*) 30
toasted (*Kretschmer*) 30
Wheat grass (*Pines*), 3 servings 29
Wheat flakes, rolled (*Arrowhead Mills*), 1/3 cup 110
Wheat flour:
all varieties, white (*Pillsbury*), 1/4 cup 100
all-purpose, white, unbleached (*Arrowhead Mills*), 1/3 cup 160
cake, white (*Swan's Down*), 1/4 cup 100
gluten (*Arrowhead Mills*), 3 tbsp. 35
pastry, soft, white, unbleached (*Arrowhead Mills*), 1/4 cup 100
pastry, soft, whole grain (*Arrowhead Mills*), 1/3 cup 100
whole grain, stone ground (*Arrowhead Mills*), 1/4 cup . . . 130
whole wheat (*Pillsbury*), 1/4 cup 120
Wheat germ:
(*Kretschmer*), 2 tbsp. 50
honey crunch (*Kretschmer*), 1 2/3 tbsp. 50
raw (*Arrowhead Mills*), 3 tbsp. 50
Wheat nuts (*Sonoma*), 2 tbsp. 60
Wheat pilaf mix (*Near East*), 1 cup* 220

Whiskey sour mixer:
bottled (*Holland House*), 4 fl. oz. 150
mix (*Bar-Tenders*), 2 pkts., 1.2 oz. 130
mix (*Bar-Tenders* Slightly Sour), 2 pkts., 1.1 oz. 120
White bean, ½ cup:
dried, boiled 125
canned, with liquid 153
canned, small (*S&W*) 80
White sauce mix (*Knorr*), ⅛ pkg., 2 tsp. 25
Whitefish, meat only, baked, broiled, or microwaved, 4 oz. 195
Whitefish, smoked, 4 oz. 122
Whiting, meat only, baked, broiled, or microwaved, 4 oz. 130
Wild rice (*Fantastic Foods*), ¼ cup 140
Wild rice dishes, see "Rice dishes, mix"
Wine, 1 fl. oz.:
dessert or apertif (sherry, port, vermouth, etc.) 41
dry or table (Burgundy, Chablis, champagne, rosé, etc.) . 25
Wine, cooking (*Holland House*), 2 tbsp.:
marsala 35
red, vermouth, or white 20
sherry 45
Wine cooler (*Bartles & Jaymes*), 12-oz. bottle:
berry, peach or strawberry 220
black cherry 210
Fuzzy Navel, Long Island iced tea, or Mai Tai 250
Margarita 270
original 200
piña colada 280
strawberry daiquiri 230
tropical 240
Winged beans, fresh, boiled, drained ½ cup 12
Winged beans, dried, boiled, ½ cup 126
Wolffish, Atlantic, meat only, baked, broiled, or microwaved, 4 oz. 139
Wonton wrapper:
(*Frieda's*), 1 piece 13
(*Nasoya*), 5 pieces, 1.2 oz. 90
Worcestershire sauce (*Lea & Perrins*), 1 tsp. 5

Y–Z

FOOD AND MEASURE	CALORIES
Yam:	
fresh, baked or boiled, ½ cup	79
canned or frozen, see "Sweet potato"	
Yam, mountain, Hawaiian, steamed, cubed, ½ cup	59
Yam bean tuber, raw (*Frieda's*), 3.5 oz.	45
Yard-long bean:	
fresh, boiled, drained, ½ cup	25
dried, boiled, ½ cup	102
Yeast, baker's, all varieties (*Fleischmann's*), ¼ tsp.	0
Yellow bean, dried, boiled, ½ cup	126
Yellow squash:	
fresh or frozen, see "Crookneck squash"	
canned (*Allen/Sunshine*), ½ cup	25
Yellowtail, meat only, baked, broiled, or microwaved, 4 oz.	212
Yogurt, 8 oz. or 1 cup, except as noted:	
plain (*Dannon* Lowfat), 8 oz.	140
plain (*Dannon* Lowfat), 1 cup	150
plain (*Dannon* Nonfat), 8 oz.	110
plain (*Dannon* Nonfat), 1 cup	120
all flavors (*Colombo* Light)	100
all flavors (*Dannon* Fruit on the Bottom)	240
all flavors (*Dannon Double Delights*), 6 oz.	170
all flavors (*Dannon Sprinkl'ins*), 4.1 oz.	140
all flavors (*Dannon Tropifruita*), 6 oz.	150
all flavors except lemon chiffon with blueberry (*Dannon Light'n Crunchy*)	150
all flavors (*Yoplait* Light), 6 oz.	90
all fruit flavors, except banana/strawberry (*Colombo* Fat Free)	200
all fruit flavors, except coconut (*Yoplait* Original Fat Free), 6 oz.	180
all fruit flavors (*Yoplait* Custard Style), 6 oz.	190

Yogurt *(cont.)*
banana cream pie or blueberry (*Dannon* Nonfat) 100
banana-strawberry or raspberry (*Colombo* Fat Free) . . . 220
cappuccino (*Colombo* Fat Free) 170
cappuccino or creme caramel (*Dannon* Nonfat) 100
cherry vanilla, strawberry, or vanilla (*Dannon* Nonfat), 8 oz. 100
coconut (*Yoplait* Original Fat Free), 6 oz. 200
coffee, lemon, or vanilla (*Dannon* Lowfat), 8 oz. 210
coffee, lemon, or vanilla (*Dannon* Lowfat), 1 cup 230
cranberry-raspberry (*Dannon* Lowfat) 210
lemon, peach, raspberry, or tropical fruit (*Dannon* Nonfat) 100
lemon chiffon with blueberry (*Dannon Light'n Crunchy*) 140
strawberry, fruit cup, or strawberry-banana (*Dannon* Nonfat) 100
vanilla (*Yoplait* Custard Style), 6 oz. 190

Yogurt, frozen, ½ cup:
all flavors (*Dannon Light'n Crunchy*) 110
all flavors, except chocolate (*Colombo* Slender Sensations/Cooler) 60
all flavors, except chocolate fudge (*Dannon Pure Indulgence*) 150
all flavors, except German chocolate fudge (*Colombo* Nonfat) 100
all flavors, except peanut butter (*Colombo* Lowfat) 110
banana pudding, homestyle (*TCBY*) 120
black cherry vanilla swirl or chocolate (*Edy's* Nonfat) 90
cappuccino (*Ben & Jerry's* Nonfat) 150
cappuccino, chocolate or vanilla (*Dannon Light*) 80
caramel praline crunch (*Edy's* Nonfat) 100
cherry vanilla, chocolate chip (*Ben & Jerry's Cherry Garcia*) 160
cherry vanilla swirl (*Dannon Light*) 90
chocolate (*Ben & Jerry's* Nonfat) 130
chocolate (*Colombo* Slender Sensations/Cooler) 70
chocolate or vanilla (*Häagen-Dazs*) 160
chocolate chip cookie dough (*Ben & Jerry's*) 210
chocolate, Dutch (*TCBY*) 100

chocolate fudge (*Dannon Pure Indulgence* Coco-Nut) . . . 160
chocolate fudge (*Edy's* Nonfat) 100
chocolate fudge, brownie (*Ben & Jerry's*) 180
chocolate fudge, German (*Colombo* Nonfat) 110
coffee fudge (*Ben & Jerry's* Nonfat) 140
coffee fudge sundae or marble fudge (*Edy's* Nonfat) . . . 100
cone crunch, crispy (*TCBY*) 130
cookies 'n cream (*TCBY*) 120
lemon chiffon or peach raspberry Melba (*Dannon Light*) 90
peach (*TCBY*) 110
peanut butter (*Colombo* Lowfat) 120
peanut butter fudge sundae or pecan praline crisp (*TCBY*) 110
pine-orange paradise, raspberry, or strawberry (*Edy's* Nonfat) 90
raspberry, black (*Ben & Jerry's* Nonfat) 140
Raspberry Rendezvous or *Strawberry Duet* (*Häagen-Dazs*) 130
strawberry cheesecake (*Dannon Light*) 90
strawberry summertime (*TCBY*) 100
toffee crunch (*Ben & Jerry's Heath*) 190
vanilla or vanilla chocolate swirl (*Edy's* Nonfat) 90
vanilla, classic (*TCBY*) 110
vanilla fudge (*Ben & Jerry's* Nonfat) 160

Yogurt bar, frozen, 1 bar:
Brownie Nut Blast (*Häagen-Dazs Exträas*) 220
cherry chocolate chip (*Ben & Jerry's Cherry Garcia*) . . . 260
cherry chocolate fudge (*Häagen-Dazs*) 240
chocolate almond (*Frozfruit* Nonfat) 130
chocolate fudge (*Edy's*) 240
peach, strawberry, or strawberry banana (*Frozfruit* Nonfat) 100
peach or raspberry and vanilla (*Häagen-Dazs*) 90
piña colada or *Tropical Orange Passion* (*Häagen-Dazs*) . . 100
(*Starburst* Lowfat), all flavors 70
Strawberry Cheesecake Craze (*Häagen-Dazs Exträas*) . . . 220
strawberry daiquiri (*Häagen-Dazs*) 90
toffee crunch (*Edy's*) 250
vanilla almond (*Edy's*) 230

Yuca, boiled, drained (*Frieda's*), 4 oz. 77
Zucchini, ½ cup, except as noted:
fresh, raw, sliced 9
fresh, baby, 1 large, 3⅛″ long, ⅝″ diameter 3
fresh, boiled, drained, sliced 14
canned, Italian style (*Del Monte*) 30
Zucchini, breaded, frozen (*Qwik-Krisp*), 6 pieces 190